MW00332319

First Blood

First Blood

A Cultural Study of Menarche

Sally Dammery

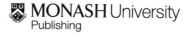

© Copyright 2016 Sally Dammery
All rights reserved. Apart from any uses permitted by Australia's Copyright
Act 1968, no part of this book may be reproduced by any process without prior
written permission from the copyright owners. Inquiries should be directed to
the publisher.

Monash University Publishing
Matheson Library and Information Services Building
40 Exhibition Walk
Monash University
Clayton, Victoria 3800, Australia
www.publishing.monash.edu

Monash University Publishing brings to the world publications which advance
the best traditions of humane and enlightened thought.

Monash University Publishing titles pass through a rigorous process of
independent peer review.

www.publishing.monash.edu/books/fb-9781925377040.html

Series: Cultural Studies

Design: Les Thomas

Cover image:
National Library of Australia Cataloguing-in-Publication entry:
Creator: Dammery, Sally, author.
Title: First blood: a cultural study of menarche / Sally
                   Dammery.
ISBN: 9781925377040 (paperback)
Notes: Includes bibliographical references and index.
Subjects: Menarche.
                   Menstruation--Cross-cultural studies.
                   Menstruation--Folklore.
                   Menstruation--Religious aspects.
Dewey Number: 305.4

Printed in Australia by Griffin Press an Accredited ISO AS/NZS 14001:2004
Environmental Management System printer.

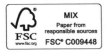

The paper this book is printed on is certified against the
Forest Stewardship Council ® Standards. Griffin Press
holds FSC chain of custody certification SGS-
COC-005088. FSC promotes environmentally
responsible, socially beneficial and economically viable
management of the world's forests.

CONTENTS

ABOUT THE AUTHOR

Sally Dammery practised clinical midwifery for many years, developing a deep interest in the diversity of cultural beliefs and traditions among the women she attended. Travelling widely increased this interest and led to formal study of anthropology and history, with later PhD research forming the basis of this book. Previous publications include the ethnography *Walter George Arthur: A Free Tasmanian?* which shared the Ian Turner History Prize in 2001, and the biography of her enigmatic grandmother, *She Lived in Launceston: Isobel Horner of Waratah House*, winner of the Lilian Watson Family History Award 2006. Sally is currently Adjunct Research Associate at the School of Philosophical, Historical and International Studies at Monash University, Australia.

ACKNOWLEDGEMENTS

This book is about an atypical subject but one familiar to young women: the first menstrual period or 'menarche'. 'The monarchy?' I have been asked, not infrequently, and then watched confusion on the faces of the questioner when I reply. So getting started was something of an obstacle course and one I look back on with considerable gratitude to those who dared take a chance and contribute in some way.

The foundation for the book lies in the willingness of the women who volunteered to participate; their interviews provided valuable primary source material and I remain profoundly grateful to them, not only for their memories shared among laughter and tears, but for their time given, and the distances they travelled to the meeting places. My gratitude also goes to the managers of the various Neighbourhood Houses and Cultural Centres who permitted me to use the facilities and who provided comfortable and quiet spaces for the interview process.

Help and support came from the School of Philosophical, Historical, and International Studies at Monash University, where David Garrioch and Marian Quartly drew my attention to certain historical reports of interest, and Mark Peel, Christina Twomey and Clare Monagle saw some potential in my early plans. From the School of Social Sciences, the anthropologists Matt Tomlinson and Brett Hough responded to my calls for help and directed me to wonderfully helpful Fijian and Indonesian women who closed the cultural gap among my interviewees.

Very special thanks to Barbara Caine who read and commented on the chapter drafts. Her admirable intellectual energy, humour and wisdom never flagged, and she deserves a special mention, as does my husband David, who provided the physical and mental space to devote to the research and writing. I am grateful, also, to Nathan Hollier and the editorial group at Monash University Publishing for their help and suggestions and also, most importantly, to the two young women who were the motivation throughout – my granddaughters.

INTRODUCTION

I remember hearing the noise, a soft jingly sound, and then, on seeing her, my surprise at how young she looked and how detached from her surroundings she seemed to be. At dawn she had been bathed and ritually dressed, each item blessed before touching her body. She wore the traditional two-piece buckskin, the buttery-coloured tunic fringed from below shoulder to wrist and decorated with symbols of the powers that would be called upon on her behalf. The skirt rippled as she walked, each of its ankle-length fringes finished with small pressed-tin cones, striking each other musically against her symbolically decorated buckskin boots. Two eagle feathers, symbols of strength, were fastened to the back of her long hair. Around her neck she wore strands of beads, including women's colours of black and white. Attached to the right side of her skirt was a drinking straw made from cattail reed, and to the left, a wooden scratching stick. Most noticeably her face had been daubed with pollen, the Apache symbol of life and renewal.[1]

The year was 1996, and the place, the ceremonial ground at the Mescalero Apache reservation in southern New Mexico where I had been invited to witness a ceremony for the young girl now walking in front of me. The reason for this important cultural occasion was female biology. She had experienced her menarche (mɛˈnɑːkɪ), a term that remains unfamiliar outside medical circles – from the Greek words mēn, meaning 'month' and arkhē, 'beginning' – her first menstrual period. She would shortly commence the deeply symbolic and ritualised activities by which she would be initiated into the knowledge of a properly lived Apache woman's life. In other words, she was to be given a pattern for living. For four days and four nights, the young girl would be attended by an older woman, her mentor, who had a specialised knowledge of the puberty ceremony. Having prepared her, this woman would continue to guide and reassure her, explaining and interpreting the classical Apache language and actions of the ceremonial practitioner – part priest, part shaman – known as a singer. For the duration of the ceremony, the girl would remain in her traditional dress, embodying the Apache cultural heroine White Painted Woman, whose ancient instruction established the rituals that celebrate a girl's menarche (the Apache language has a separate naming term for this event, indicating its cultural significance). Although the

---

1   Author's journal (unpublished), 'Apache Puberty Ceremony 4–7 July 1996', Mescalero
     Apache Reservation, New Mexico USA.

wider community is involved in this celebration, the major focus is on the ceremonial subject, the girl, believed at this time to have the dual powers of healing and destruction. While her ability to meet the needs of many others would be tested by demands for her touch, to bless and to heal, the same touch under other conditions was thought to be potentially destructive. Hence the cattail drinking straw, fastened to her skirt, to prevent her coming in contact with water, an act which was traditionally believed to cause destructive rains and floods. Similarly, the scratching stick to relieve itches prevented her destructive touch scarring her own body. These aspects of Apache belief about menarche are not magnified, and the general impression one gets from watching the ceremony is of good-humoured support by the onlookers and a sense of achievement by the girl in having officially reached the status of young woman.[2]

Much has been written about the Apache puberty ceremony and observing it added another dimension to my understanding of the cultural differences I increasingly encountered, both in my work as a hospital-based midwife and in my anthropological and historical studies. From time to time the media reports that menarche is occurring at a younger age in the Western world, paralleling increasing obesity in children.[3] I read about it and vaguely considered the social implications, and then something happened that brought me into direct contact with the subject. My granddaughter, a ten year-old wisp of a girl, new to the state and to her school, and with no established circle of friends, had her first period. Knowing that determinants of age at menarche included genetic and environmental factors, and situations of psychological stress, it was understandable.[4]

2   For a detailed study of this complex ceremony see 'The girl's puberty rite', in anthropologist Morris E. Opler, *An Apache Life-Way: the Economic, Social, and Religious Institutions of the Chiricahua Indians*, Cooper Square Publishers Inc., New York 1965, pp. 82–134. First published by the University of Chicago Press, 1941, this remains a key text. See also anthropologist Claire R. Farrer's interesting interpretation of the ceremony, 'Singing for life', in *Living Life's Circle: Mescalero Apache Cosmovision*, University of New Mexico Press, Albuquerque 1991, pp. 128–183 and Henrietta H. Stockel's descriptive, 'The Puberty Ceremony' in *Chiricahua Women and Children: Safekeepers of the Heritage*, Texas A&M University Press, College Station 2000, pp. 33–40.

3   Nicole Brady 'Puberty blues: the trials of young girls growing up faster than ever', *The Sunday Age*, 22 May 2011, pp. 4–5. Popular opinion is that the age of menarche has fallen significantly in Australia although paediatric and adolescent gynaecologist Julie Quinlivan, cited in Brady's article, gives the average age as 12 years and 7 months. See also the editorial in the same edition, 'Tending to children with the bodies of women', p. 14.

4   James S. Chisholm, Julie A. Quinlivan, Rodney W. Petersen, David A. Coall, 'Early stress predicts age at menarche and first birth, adult attachment, and expected

Her mother had also experienced early menarche and had explained the biological event in preparation but that was then, and this was the reality. Adding to the difficulties was the lack of primary school infrastructure to cater to menstruating girls so there were no pads or bins in the toilets, and her teacher was a stranger she felt unable to confide in. Consequently, her menarche was an alarming, lonely, and negative experience.

Reflecting on these two events resulted in more questions. Where do ideas associated with first periods come from? Where might cultural differences have originated? Who is responsible for the construction and why? Does the onset of the menstrual cycle influence how women will live their lives? I had been allowed a glimpse of an alternative way to think of menarche in the Apache ceremony, but was it unique to Apaches? Australia is home to women of many different cultures. What were their experiences, particularly older immigrant women from countries without the culture-flattening effects of television? Had any undergone some form of ceremony? More importantly, might my findings be of help to pre-adolescent girls, particularly recent immigrants from non-English-speaking backgrounds, whose cultural beliefs about menarche and menstruation might enhance their feelings of alienation?

These questions formed the beginning of a research study based on a series of unstructured interviews with English-speaking immigrant women of 50 years and over. An initial outreach to colleagues who I'd known well over many years made me aware of two important issues: the reticence women feel being asked to speak of deeply private matters outside a doctor's consulting room or a hospital, and the cultural silence on matters related to menstruation customary among many ethnic groups, including Chinese women. Ultimately, however, 54 interviews took place with women whose native countries included Greece, Italy, Lebanon, Ukraine, England, Uganda, Sri Lanka, India, Fiji, Chile, Singapore, Hong Kong, Vietnam, Korea, Philippines and Indonesia. (Their real names have been replaced by culturally appropriate others).

As the interviews progressed, certain repeated themes became apparent and eventually formed the subject of each chapter. These themes, clearly identified, included the immediate response to menarche; the concept of

---

lifespan', *Human Nature*, vol. 16, no. 3, 2005, pp. 236-238. See also Scott Dickson and Ruth Wood, 'The perceptions, experiences and meanings rural girls ascribe to menarche: implications for teachers/teachers in training', paper presented at the Australian Association for Research in Education Conference, Hobart 1995, http://www.aare.edu.au/95pap/dicks95021.txt

being 'dirty'; menstrual stories or myths heard at menarche; the menarche ceremony; the fear of revealing menstrual bleeding and how concealment was achieved; and the almost total ignorance of menstrual knowledge. Although my original intention was to construct a cultural history of menarche, the emergent themes opened up issues outside historical scholarship. Cultural history in the construction of meaning associated with menarche would not be ignored, but it was inadequate for this particular work.

Consequently, a study of medical, religious, philosophical and anthropological discourses surrounding menarche was necessary for me to provide both a framework and context for interpretation of the interview data. This broad literature helped me to identify the way in which meanings were constructed in many cultures, and also where similarities and differences were situated. Increasingly, too, it became important for readers that the book commence with an overview of historical attitudes and beliefs about blood. This is intended to enable an understanding of the foundational sources of knowledge about menarche and menstruation, the major influences on how women's bodies and blood were understood, and the accumulation and changing focus of knowledge.

So although menarche and menstruation are shared biological phenomena with deeper investigation revealing certain past commonalities of cultural meanings, scientific knowledge and progress continue to supplant cultural traditions, and different ways of thought about the body and its cyclical bleeding continue to emerge.

Chapter 1

OF BLOOD AND BLEEDING

In the introduction, two very different instances of the same physiological event were presented. One was a public celebration of a private experience, the other a miserably lonely private discovery. The public ceremony was part of indigenous culture and the private recognition reflected the Anglo-Australian tradition of learned silence surrounding bodily processes beyond infancy and early childhood. In both cases, the common factor was bleeding. Therefore, before the voices of the interviewees are introduced I want to provide an overview of the major historical influences that shape ideas about blood, particularly the blood of menarche and menstruation. This will enable a wider understanding of statements made by interviewees from predominantly non-English-speaking backgrounds, whose experiences of menarche pre-date access to knowledge through electronic technology and social media.

Outside of the medical sciences, what do we know about blood and bleeding? This word blood, with its female connotations, arises from Nordic and Saxon through Old English, and relates to women's domestic environment and their emotions. It is a word invoking the way in which we think of our bodies, from the earliest childhood horror of a bleeding cut to the adult dread of the bleeding disease, Ebola. Universally we learn that blood is part of life, invisible within the body boundaries, and that its visibility signifies injury or disease and perhaps even death. Menarche, therefore, is a paradox. It is uniquely a blood loss associated with health and an indicator of potential life, yet its meaning has in many ways been constructed in opposition to the reality.

Western understanding of blood and bleeding began in Classical Greece, with the most significant scholars of human physiology being the Hippocratics and Aristotle. The Hippocratics were a diverse group, most of whom practised medicine, although not necessarily of Hippocrates' school or even within Hippocrates' lifetime. They wrote over a lengthy time span, from the second half of the fifth century to the mid-fourth century BCE, contributing to a corpus of approximately 60 treatises, of which 10 are gynaecological.[1] Their knowledge and understanding of the body and its processes was constructed without dissection but with certain extrapolations from animal carcasses. As a result the Hippocratics believed women's bodies were made up of mammary-like glands, spongy and absorbent, capable of soaking up and retaining far more fluid than male bodies, and that this moistness characterised the principal difference between the sexes.[2] They constructed ideas of women's internal processes through observation of external mammary and menstrual signs; their theories of menstrual blood consistency, amount and duration were shaped by existing societal ideas of women.[3]

Menarche, according to the Hippocratics, confirmed the closing stages of puberty. Until then they considered girls to be similar to boys. Physiologically, the bodily changes in a young girl were thought to be caused by significantly increased blood made from food intake during the early adolescent growth spurt. When this ceased, and less activity was undertaken, it became an excess to be evacuated through the lower internal structures of uterus or womb. As a result, the menarcheal girl's body was, as classicist Lesley Dean-Jones suggests, a newly completed system of blood-hydraulics, continuously generating and discharging blood throughout reproductive life; the attached social meaning was that menarche visibly signalled the end of childhood.[4] One of the three writers of the Hippocratic gynaecological treatise 'Diseases of Women' theorised the moment of menarche began when the veins supplying the uterus widened sufficiently to enable blood to actually flow.[5]

As a result of that moment, the young girl began to bleed, metaphorically paralleling ritual Greek animal sacrifice, in which blood that clotted quickly indicated good health in the animal and augured well for the health of the community. The Hippocratics believed clotting in menstrual blood indicated good health also, and Dean-Jones argues a sacrificial connotation to the menarcheal girl, who might now renew the body civic as well as her

---

1   Lesley Dean-Jones, *Women's Bodies in Classical Greek Science* (1994), Oxford
     University Press, Oxford 2001, pp. 7, 10. See also Luigi Arata, 'Menses in the corpus
     Hippocraticum', in *Menstruation: a Cultural History*, Andrew Shail and Gillian Howie
     (eds), Palgrove Macmillan, Basingstoke 2005, p. 13.
2   Dean-Jones (2001), p. 55.
3   Lesley Dean-Jones, 'Menstrual bleeding according to the Hippocrates and Aristotle',
     Transactions of the American Philological Association, vol. 119, 1989, p. 177–178.
4   Dean-Jones, (2001), pp. 46–55, 225, 229.
5   Arata in Shail and Howie (eds) (2005), p. 15.

own.[6] Understandably, problems arose if a girl passed 14 without beginning to menstruate, and this was taken to mean an obstruction to the passages. The girl's health was thought to become compromised by the ever-increasing dangerous waste sealed inside her body, which would rise to the area around the heart, causing change to sensation and progressing to symptoms akin to epilepsy and finally causing potential suicide.[7] The treatment for this perilous situation is prescribed in a text from the Hippocratic *On the Diseases of Virgins:*

> Relief from this complaint comes when nothing impedes the flow of blood. I order parthenoi to marry as quickly as possible if they suffer this. For if they become pregnant, they will become healthy.[8]

Classicist Helen King examines the social and cultural context in which the Hippocratics constructed their ideas about women's bodies. King considers that the problem of a non-bleeding young girl might be more her resistance to social pressure to marry and reproduce rather than her symptoms.[9] A slightly different perspective is taken by classicist Helen Demand, who suggests that the cultural construction of early marriage as the cure for symptoms might have served to reconcile the girl to premature defloration at a time when fear and apprehension were attributes valued in brides by men.[10] So although we understand the treatment to be within the parameters of social expectation we cannot know how the girl, as subject, responded. Her menarche, an intensely private event, would become a shared endeavour achieved belatedly through male intervention, by physician or husband, with her defloration and marriage accelerating the transition from the young, single but marriageable *parthenos*, to adult woman or *gynê*, which a first birth completed. Yet another diagnosis was that of blood trapped in immature, narrow blood vessels. The treatment for this was applications of warmth to dilate the vessels and bring about menarche.[11] Assisting girls to bleed was significant in Classical Greek

---

6   Dean-Jones (1989), p. 191.
7   Dean-Jones (2001), pp. 19, 46–55.
8   Hippocrates, *On the Diseases of Virgins* (L8.466-71) cited in Helen King, *Hippocrates' Woman: Reading the Female Body in Ancient Greece,* Routledge, London 1998, p. 78. See also Hippocrates, 'Girls', in *Hippocrates, Vol. IX,* trans. Paul Potter (ed.), Loeb Classical Library, Harvard University Press, Cambridge (US) 2010, pp. 259–263.
9   King (1998), p.79.
10   Nancy H. Demand, 'Acculturation to Early Childhood', in *Birth, Death and Motherhood in Classical Greece,* The Johns Hopkins University Press, Baltimore 1994, p. 103.
11   Dean Jones (2001), pp. 50–51; King (1998), p. 77.

society. Men might shed blood in battle but girls bled to become women in menarche, menstruation, defloration and childbirth.[12]

Contrasting with the Hippocratics, Aristotle wrote as a sole author in the latter part of the fourth century BCE, adding to and adapting his biological theories over the years. He believed the physiological difference between men and women was female menstruation, and reasoned the monthly flow caused the body temperature in women to be cooler than in men. However, Aristotle, whose template of the human was male, qualified what he means by 'women':

> Everything reaches its perfection sooner in females than in males – e.g. puberty, maturity, old age – because females are weaker and colder in their nature; and we should look upon the female state as being as it were a deformity, though one which occurs in the ordinary state of nature.[13]

Aristotle believed puberty began at 14, when menarche initiated the transition from girl to woman without confirming readiness for the adult role.[14] He observes that female puberty was signalled by voice change, as in the male, and by breast development.[15] Both semen and menstrual blood were thought to be residue from purified nourishment, but discharged menstrual blood was useless according to Aristotle, because it was fluid.[16] In matters of reproduction Aristotle believed both men and women embodied the 'principle' of generation. The heat of the male body 'concocted' semen to contain the principle of 'form' or 'soul', the essence of a particular body.[17] Females lacked the heat to 'concoct' and their colder bodies and narrower blood vessels prevented them from storing any over-supply of nourishment. Menstruation, therefore, was the excess and was inclined to occur with the waning moon at the colder time of the month.[18] At conception, the female provided the material from menstrual fluid contained in the uterus, which semen acted upon in a similar manner to rennet setting warm milk, giving rise to the belief that menstrual fluid and milk were essentially identical. Once 'set', foetal growth was dependent on maternal blood from the uterine wall via the umbilical cord.[19]

---

12   King (1998), p. 84.
13   Aristotle, *Generation of Animals XIII*, trans. A. L. Peck (1942), Loeb Classical Library, William Heinemann Limited, London 1963, pp. 460–461.
14   Dean-Jones (2001), p. 53.
15   Aristotle, *Generation*, 726b, 727a, p. 95.
16   Aristotle, *Generation*, 725a, 739a, pp. 81, 187.
17   Aristotle, *Generation*, 731b, 738b, 765b, pp. 129, 185, 385.
18   Aristotle, *Generation*, 738a, p. 181.
19   Aristotle, *Generation*, 727b, 739b, 740a, pp. 101, 191, 193, 197.

Although medical practitioners were socially placed to be influential observers of women, that is, to help shape social practice regarding women, classicist M.K. Hopkins emphasises that their patients were more likely to come from upper socio-economic groups of their communities – those who could afford their fees.[20] One such physician was Soranus, who had studied in Alexandria and practised in Rome in the early second century CE. He is remembered for his writings, including on gynaecology, and his methods of treatment were still being used into the 16th century due to continuing translation and compilation of his texts. Soranus' ideas of women's bodies and of menarche are interesting, not only because he learned through human dissection but because they allow comparison with the earlier Hippocratics.[21] His observation of menarche is that it occurs 'at the time of puberty', rather than as its completion, as the Hippocratics believed. The age of menarche is 'around the fourteenth year', indicating recognition of individual variation, and the same principle is applied to the menstrual cycle, allowing a slight difference between women in cyclical timing but with regularity within the variation. Soranus refutes the notion that a waning moon influenced the start of menstruation and observed the amount of blood loss was affected by seasonal change, body weight and physical activity with a maximum of two cotyles, about 450 mls, also considered normal by the Hippocratics. Anaemia would seem a likely outcome until we remember that women were pregnant or lactating from a very early age, hence not bleeding, for a great part of their menstrual lives. Soranus believed in preparation of girls, at about 13, in advance of defloration. He recommended a form of pelvic rocking through passive swinging, together with walking, being massaged and bathed daily and being mentally occupied. For Soranus a relaxed mind and body encouraged an unproblematic menarche and puberty and he writes, 'even if the body be changed for the better, all abruptness disturbs it through discomfort'. His ideas about the purpose of menarche-menstruation are not dissimilar from the excretory notions of the Hippocratics and Aristotle. He defines the purpose of the uterus as threefold: menstruation, conception and pregnancy. Soranus reasons menstrual blood 'is useful for childbearing only' as it becomes food for the embryo, otherwise it is excreted as 'excessive matter', beginning with menarche at about 14, signalling 'this age then is

---

20 M. K. Hopkins, 'The age of Roman girls at marriage', *Population Studies*, vol. 18, no. 3, 1965, p. 312.

21 Owsei Temkin, 'Introduction', in Soranus, *Gynaecology*, trans. Owsei Temkin (1956), The Johns Hopkins University Press, Baltimore 1991, pp. xxiii, xxv. See also Soranus, p. 15.

really the natural one indicating the time for defloration'.[22] In this, Soranus warns against the hazards of childbirth that premature defloration could cause. He strongly believed that menarche and defloration should occur together but that menarche should precede marriage.[23]

As we have seen, the age of menarche assumed great social significance in Classical Greece and Rome. Hopkins studied the average age of Roman girls at menarche citing the hypothesis of M. Durry, who extrapolated from work in North Africa that pre-pubescent marriage occurred among the Romans, that puberty was irrelevant to fixing an age of marriage and that marriage was consummated before menarche. Hopkins counters that although Rome c.400 CE had commonalities with the modern Western family, Roman understanding of marriage was dissimilar from that of today.[24]

Soranus wrote that menarche occurred at about 14. Not unreasonably, Hopkins queries whether girls from all social strata have been represented, pointing out the trend towards earlier menarche among the upper socio-economic group, with their smaller families and adequate nourishment, compared with manual workers. He notes that studies of 19th-century Europe reveal a menarcheal age difference of two years between the two groups. Yet later Roman marriage laws, from the time of Augustus to about 530 CE, made 12 the legal age of marriage for girls, providing another complication to the accepted age of menarche. Does this mean an earlier menarche had become generalised or that Rome condoned pre-menarcheal marriage? Hopkins points out that the men girls married were considerably older and not necessarily known to them. One example is the daughter of Emperor Claudius, Octavia, who married at 11, although according to Roman lawyer Julian, marriage under 12 constituted engagement, regardless of the formalities, until the legal age was reached. When we read of family alliances being made and dowries being specified, the socio-economic reasons for the early marriage of girls become clearer. Soranus' warning about early defloration and his exercises aimed at making a premature experience less traumatic both suggest that consummated pre-menarcheal marriage was not unknown.[25]

---

22   *Soranus,* trans. Temkin (1991), pp. 16–19, 21–22, 27, 31. For the Hippocratic menstrual blood loss ideal see Dean-Jones (1989), p. 180.
23   Hopkins (1965), p. 314.
24   Hopkins (1965), p. 309-310.
25   Hopkins (1965), pp. 312–316, 327.

At the time of the Classical Greeks and Romans, other ideas about women's bodies, menarche and menstruation were being constructed in China and India. Once again, the writers of surviving data were practitioners of medicine and, as social scientist and historian Michel Foucault observes, the physician's gaze varies according to shifts in parameters of bodily orientation in differing historical periods.[26] The same may be said of differing cultures and beliefs about women's bodies.

In an explanation and commentary on Chinese medicine, medical researcher Ted K. Kaptchuk explains that the *Huang Di Nei Jing*, or Inner Classic of the Yellow Emperor (known as Nei Jing), are the oldest Chinese medical texts and the equivalent of the Hippocratic corpus, compiled by unknown male writers between 300 and 100 BCE.[27] Chinese understanding of physiology is based on fundamental substances which include qi, blood and jing. Underlying these fundamentals is the idea of yin and yang, complementary opposition. They are neither forces, nor material beings, but systems of thought in which all things are part of a continuously changing whole.[28] Blood is a yin substance and the end-process of food transformed by qi, a yang substance, which is then transported through the body by heart qi. Blood has close relationships with heart, liver and spleen, but is indissoluble from qi which creates, moves and holds it in place. In medieval China, blood was thought to be carried through blood vessels and meridians, the pathways being considered of less importance than the function.[29] Meridians are not blood vessels but conceptual conduits symbolising a physical reality, carrying qi and blood through the body, regulating yin and yang, and linking all vital substances and organs.[30] According to Kaptchuk, qi is sometimes translated

---

26 Michel Foucault, *The Birth of the Clinic: an Archaeology of Medical Perception*, trans. A. M. Sheridan Smith, Vintage Books, New York, 1994, p. 54.

27 Ted J. Kaptchuk, *Chinese Medicine: the Web that has no Weaver*, (1983), Rider and Company, Essex 1987, p.23. Nei Jing was the foundation of later Chinese medical theories and commentaries, which evolved into those of the Han Dynasty (200 BCE–200 CE), the Ming Dynasty (1368–1645) and the Qing Dynasty (1644–1911).

28 Kaptchuck (1987), pp. 7–8.

29 Kaptchuk (1987), p. 41.

30 Kaptchuk (1987), pp. 7–8, 77–78. The term 'meridian' entered the English language from the French translation for the Chinese 'jing-luo', 'jing' meaning 'to go through' or 'thread in a fabric' and 'Luo' meaning 'something that connects or attaches' or 'a net'. See p. 77. The term is not without its critics. Paul Unschuld, translator and commentator of the ancient Chinese medical texts, *Huang Di nei jing su wen*, argues 'meridian' is a term widely used in Western acupuncture writings and which fails to parallel the salient 'jing' concept. Unschuld believes Western use of the term is a construction removed from historical fact. See note 382 in 'Notes', p. 370, Paul U. Unschuld, *Huang Di nei jing su wen: Nature, Knowledge, Imagery in an Ancient Chinese Medical Text*, University of California Press, Berkely and Los Angeles, 2003.

as vital energy, but energy in Chinese thought is not distinguishable from matter. Qi, therefore, could be considered as matter on the brink of becoming energy, or vice-versa.[31] The third fundamental substance is jing, which Kaptchuk defines as the essence of all organic life and organic transformation. Understood as fluid, jing is the source of reproduction and development: firstly as the prenatal inheritance from parents, determining growth and development, and secondly as a postnatal source derived from ingested food, which, once purified, provides prenatal jing with vitality to balance growth with energy, a process that moves through seven-year stages.[32]

In ancient China the uterus, known literally as 'palace of the child', is considered to be a curious, or peculiar, organ – yang in form, because it disperses rather than stores, but yin in function, storing rather than dispersing. Its functionality is subsumed under primary organs or meridians. As a result, menarche and menstruation cannot occur without the governing function of other organs, the liver, spleen or kidneys together with a conception and penetrating meridian, both thought to arise in the uterus.[33] Thus, the *Nei Jing* states that women's bodies develop in seven-year stages and the significance attached to the second stage, at 14, is the arrival of the jing Dew of Heaven, or menarche. In her study on gender in China's medical history, Charlotte Furth points out that the menarcheal age, given as 14, is the age in sui, that is, calculated from conception. Menarche, then, was socially anticipated at 13 – but what did ancient Chinese believe menstruation was?

Menstruation was seen by early medieval Chinese physicians as a diagnostic guide to women's internal body processes and general physiological condition according to Sabine Wilms. Medical practitioners believed that 'in women, one first regulates Blood, in men, one first regulates qi'.[34] Menstrual blood told the story of reproductive health and process. It was believed to nourish the foetus in pregnancy, then travel and transform to

---

31   Kaptchuk (1987), p. 35.
32   Kaptchuk (1987), p. 43.
33   Kaptchuck (1987), pp.43, 336–337, 'Appendix F: the Curious Organs'. See also Furth (1999), p. 45.
34   Chen Zeming, juan 6, 175, cited in Sabine Wilms, 'The art and science of menstrual balancing in early medieval China', in *Menstruation: a Cultural History*, Andrew Shail and Gillian Howie (eds), Palgrave Macmillan, Basingstoke 2005, p. 39. Chen Zeming (1190–1270) was a 'fuke' or what we would term gynaecologist, and author of *All-inclusive Good Prescriptions for Women (Furen ta quan liang fang)* compiled in 1237 and published in 1284. See also Charlotte Furth, *A Flourishing Yin: Gender in China's Medical History, 960–1665*, University of California Press, Berkeley and Los Angeles, 1999, p. 70.

milk in lactation. Any blockage in the channels of transport were cause for concern, consequently a regular and copious flow reflected blooming health and balance.[35] In this, Wilms could be describing the Hippocratics; so could the influential physician Sun Simiao, c.561–662 CE, who wrote of girls:

> From the age of fourteen [sui] on, their yin qi wells up and a hundred thoughts run through their minds, damaging their organ systems within and ruining their beauty without. Their monthly courses flow out or are retained within, now early, now late, stagnating and congesting Blood and interrupting the functions of central pathways. The injuries from this cannot be enumerated in words.[36]

At the time Sun wrote, the practice of medicine as 'impersonal, constant, and rule governed'[37] was confined to court in the imperial capital, and by no means representative of the many states. There are echoes with Classical Greece in written perceptions of girls and women and in the medicalisation of the menarcheal and menstrual process within the urban setting. Although the court had its share of women healers, according to Furth, we have no access to accounts by women of their experiences.[38] We do know, however, that during the Song dynasty female desire was problematic in regard to puberty. There was concern about the effects of shifting balances of bodily forces on delicate girls' bodies not yet ready for birthing, as signified by blushing. The influence of fifth-century CE court physician Chu Cheng, whom Furth maintains was somewhat of an early eugenicist, resulted in social proscription of sexual knowledge for a decade post-puberty, followed by marriage without delay. The exception was among upper-class girls, who continued to marry at a young age.[39] As a result, the bodies of young women who lived in communities such as the Imperial Court were protected by the growing medical interest in their physiological conditions, which included reproductive capabilities, beginning at menarche.

India is the site of Ayurveda, the other great tradition in historic constructions of women's blood and bodies, a system of ancient medical teachings believed to have been introduced to India in the time of the Buddha, c.450 BCE. In his translation and notes on the text, medical historian and Sanskrit scholar Dominik Wujastyk considers Ayurveda to be significant in

---

35   Wilms (2005), pp. 38–39.
36   Sun Simiao, *Prescriptions Worth a Thousand (Beiji qianjin yaofang)* quoted in Furth (1999), p. 71.
37   Unschuld (2003), p. 320.
38   Furth (1999), pp. 60–61, 67.
39   Furth (1999), pp. 53, 89–90.

many ways, one being the evolution of a unified set of ideas and practices from the many in existence. Written in Sanskrit by scholarly men, these texts formed the fundamental learning texts for the formal study of medicine, and they remain so today, supported by the Indian government.[40] Central to the Ayurvedic construct of the body is digestion, or transformation of food into a vital essence known as rasa, which has some similarity with the Chinese concept of jing. There are two different texts that describe the attributes of rasa. In Suśruta's *Compendium*, rasa moves through the body and, in an oppositional process reminiscent of yin and yang, drinks from the cooling fluid principle of Soma. When rasa meets the fiery principle contained in the kidneys and spleen, the fluid becomes reddened and, in women, transforms into menstrual blood. Therefore, menstrual blood is of a fiery principle. Thus:

> The pure water in people's bodies is dyed (rañjita) by the clear, fiery principle which is present in the body. For this reason it is called blood (rakta). A woman's blood, which issues from the same nutritive juice, is termed 'menstrual blood'. It starts in the twelfth year.[41]

The authorities who wrote the alternative version have blood formed through the shared principle of the five elements: earth, water, fire, air and space, characterised by a raw odour, fluidity, red colour, pulsation and lightness respectively. According to Wujastyk this version is not elaborated in the text, which returns to blood creation by a process of transubstantiation from purified digestive material that has become rasa. Blood is the first of the body matters to be generated, transubstantiating to flesh, and continuing until the final essence, that of semen, over the course of a cycle that takes one lunar month. Having argued there is no female equivalent, Wujastyk's translation later positions menstrual blood as an end product parallel to semen, giving evidence of some recognised inconsistency in the texts.[42]

The Ayurvedic fables are cautionary tales built around a demoness and child-killer, Lady Opulence. They are contained in Kaśyapa's *Compendium*, c. first millennium BCE, which advises on diseases of women and children

---

40   Dominik Wujastyk, *The Roots of Ayurveda*, Penguin Books Limited (1998), London, 2003, pp. xv–xvi.
41   Suśruta's *Compendium*, trans. Dominik Wujastyk in Wujastyk (2003), p. 110. Wujastyk has difficulty identifying the time of Suśruta's work, arguing that the latest possible date for the text would be 600 CE, but also that possible reference was made to him through a grammatical rule in c. 250 BCE.
42   Wujastyk (2003), pp. xix. See also Suśruta in Wujastyk pp. 72–73, 111 f.n. 59. Suśruta is the oldest surviving manuscript today, written by scholars over a lengthy period commencing c 250 BCE with a final editing c sixth-century CE. See pp. 63–64.

and are intended as explanations for miscarriage and infant or child death, based on the notion that disease is due to evil conduct. One example is:

> If a woman has not started to menstruate by the time she is sixteen, if her arms are scrawny and she has no breasts, then she is said to be 'Parched Lady Opulence'.

This seems like a harsh labelling for a girl who might already be suffering socially from her absent menarche. Kaśyapa calls such young girls destroyers of menstruation and pronounces them incurable.[43] We are not told their fate and there is nothing more about menarche in the translated texts. I believe the significance of this fable lies in the girl's age and physical description, possibly caused by existing famine or disease.

Returning to Europe, the medieval era in Italy brought forward the mysterious Trotula, who lived in Salerno, about the 11th or 12th century CE. The authoritative Latin text *On the Diseases of Women* is attributed to her, as is her position as first female professor of medicine at Salerno. But is it all myth? Medical historian Monica H. Green writes that there were three texts, two anonymous, probably from Salerno, and one (the second, *On Treatments for Women*) thought to have come be written by Trota, a woman midwife or healer. The three texts were compiled into one late in the 12th century and titled *Trotula*, meaning 'little Trota'. According to Green, the texts are significant because they demonstrate developing the theories on women's physiology and the spreading influence of Arabic medicine in Europe, as well as giving indications of how women understood themselves and their bodies within the medical framework of the time.[44] Medical historian Charles Singer is scathing, relegating Trotula to the English nursery as Dame Trot and arguing that Trottus was a male doctor at Salerno whose collected works, of origins far earlier than the Middle Ages, were known as the Trotula. Singer maintains that the content of the work suggests a male author with a propensity for invasion of the private female space.[45]

---

43 Kaśyapa's *Compendium*, trans. Wujastyk in Wujastyk (2003), pp. 165–166; 175–176. Kaśyapa's *Compendium* remains fragmentary. It was written on palm leaves and the first of the surviving two texts was discovered in Katmandu in 1898. Because of the archaic language the writing is believed to be first millennium BCE. See pp. 165–166.

44 *The Trotula: a Medieval Compendium of Women's Medicine*, trans. Monica H. Green (ed.), University of Pennsylvania Press, Philadelphia, 2001, p. xi–xiii.

45 Charles Singer, *From Magic to Science*, Dover, New York, 1958, p. 244. The nursery rhyme is as follows: 'Dame Trot and her cat had a peaceable life when they were not troubled by other folks' strife: when Dame had her dinner pussy would wait and was sure to receive a nice piece from her plate'. According to The Shorter Oxford English

Trotula's woman is cold and moist, a combination of the Hippocratic and the Aristotelian, with reference made to the Hippocratics. Increasingly weak, she is a victim of repeated pregnancies and gynaecological disease. Her menarche, or 'flowers' as people referred to menstruation, occurred at about 13 years, and the timing is attributed to her body heat or coldness.[46] However, Green asserts that since age given for medieval menarche is prescribed, it is historically unreliable, although she also refers to a 15th-century Dutch translation of Trotula which states 'and it comes to some at their sixteenth years and to some at their ninth year', indicating considerable variation existed.[47] Trotula's explanation for menstruation is that women lack the heat to dry out bodily fluid for excretion as sweat, in the manner of men. Their innate weakness prevents them labouring sufficiently hard to create enough heat, thus menstruation compensates, recurring regularly to empty out waste. Like the Hippocratics, Trotula regards a heavy blood flow as cleansing and synonymous with health but associates irregularity in flow with sickness.[48]

In late medieval England the influence of the Christian church brought about a shift in conceptualising the lives of young girls who, under medieval canon law, reached the age of consent at 12,[49] the age when the Virgin Mary experienced her menarche.[50] Symbolised as the Virgin Mother of Jesus Christ, representations of Mary in text and image depicted her as beautiful young woman and served to popularise the model of maidenhood as a virtue.[51] Maidenhood was, according to historian Kim M. Phillips, the perfect age in

---

Dictionary, third edition (1944), C.T. Onions (ed.), Oxford 1959, p. 1627, pussy, as applied to girl or woman entered the English lexicon about 1583, so the provenance of the rhyme would be of interest to explore in the historical context.

46   *Trotula*, trans. Green (ed.) (2001), pp. 71, 73.

47   *Trotula*, trans. Green (ed.) (2001), note 85, p. 215. The quote is from Anna Delva, *Vrouwengeneeskunde in Vlaanderen tijdens de late middeleeuwen*, Brugge: Vlaamse Historische Studies, 1983, p. 162.

48   *Trotula*, trans. Green (ed.) (2001), pp. 71, 73, 75.

49   Kim M. Phillips, 'Maidenhood as the perfect age of woman's life', in *Young Medieval Women*, Katherine J. Lewis, Noël James Menuge and Kim M. Phillips (eds), Sutton Publishing Limited, Gloucestershire, 1999, pp. 1, 4. Phillips refers to the term 'maiden' as being in use late 1300s to 1500 CE, pp. 1, 2, 4, 5, 16.

50   Charles T. Wood, 'The doctor's dilemma: sin, salvation and the menstrual cycle in medieval thought', *Speculum*, vol. 56, no. 4, 1981, p. 722. Wood cites *The Protevangelium of James, New Testament Apocrypha*, Wilhelm Schneemelcher (ed.), R. McL. Wilson (tr.), as the source of this quotation. An internet search gave an alternative 1886 translation by Alexander Roberts, James Donaldson and Arthur C. Coxe. See *The Infancy Gospel of James*, 8:2, http:// www.earlychristianwritings.com/text/infancyjames-roberts.html as verification. Janice Delaney, Mary Jane Upton and Emily Toth also include reference to the menarche of the Virgin Mary in *The Curse: a Cultural History of the Menstruation*, (1976,) University of Illinois Press, Urbana, 1988, p. 40.

51   Phillips in Lewis et al (1999), pp. 4, 12.

a woman's life, representing an idealised state of femininity, a concept widely popularised by a male elite, including members of the clergy, who generated representations of virginal perfection beginning at menarche when the young girl was neither child nor woman.[52] This stage in her life-cycle could be from the age of between 12 to 15 until late-teens to mid-20s, when marriage in England was more likely to take place. However, Phillips acknowledges that marriage preceding canonical age took place among some of the upper classes and gentry, driven by socio-political or economic interests, albeit with the recognition of a lost phase of maidenhood.[53] Phillips also raises two separate issues: she makes a brief reference to food shortage in the mid-14th century without associating it with a later onset of menarche, and she places the common and borough legal age of majority as mid-teen, which suggests the two may be linked. A third situation is the institution of service, through participation in cloistered life, by many girls from their mid-teens to mid-20s, which was recognised and accommodated in English culture.[54] This state of maidenhood provoked certain tensions between maturation and the preservation of virginity until marriage, and is, Phillips considers, fundamental to the concept of feminine identity in late-medieval England. Legends evolved from the construction of the idealised courageous maiden defending her chastity against the attentions of the villainous pagan suitor. Examples of virgin martyrs proliferated. Their shared attributes were their menarcheal age, their beauty and their sexual appeal, and all had pledged their virginity to God at a time of their life that Phillips believes represents the female version of Aristotle's 'perfect manhood'.[55]

Literary use of names and terms enables us to trace other changes in social thought. We have an example of male attitude towards menarche in the 1600s in Milton's Trinity manuscript, *A Mask*, in which Comus, the male suitor of the maiden Lady, refers to her 'lees'. The interpreter, B.J. Sokol, uses the framework of the Lady's menarche as the context for dialogue between the two. Comus is a metaphor for the pagan and the Lady is the non-acquiescent virgin. Comus speaks of 'tilted lees' and 'settlings of a melancholy blood' using the fermentation theory of menstruation and denigrating the Lady through inference that menstruation affects behaviour and detracts from desirability. He receives his come-uppance from the Lady, whose words he suggests have come from 'some superior power'. Sokol argues this to be a

---

52   Phillips in Lewis et al (1999), p. 5, 16.
53   Phillips in Lewis et al (1999), pp. 4–5.
54   Phillips in Lewis et al (1999), pp. 4, 5, 8.
55   Phillips in Lewis et al (1999), pp. 5, 10, 11.

moral victory amid the turbulence of menarche, and one that shows Milton may have been influenced by shifting ideas about menstruation. At the time there was some revisionist medical thought that menarche and menstruation were sickening conditions only when illness already existed. Yet, as Dean-Jones has noted, Aristotle viewed menstruation as a normal part of a woman's life without any thought of pollution to be taken into account. Sokol continues the thesis that menarche is both a serious and significant event transforming the girl-child to the marriageable virgin, and going so far as to suggest Milton's masque might well have been a clandestine celebration of menarche in which the maiden, as a young, beautiful and sexually alluring virgin, is accepted into the community as ready and able to enter marriage and thus lose her virginity.[56]

By the close of the 1600s, women were asking what menstrual blood really was, as historian Cathy McClive has shown in her research into menstrual knowledge in early modern France. A midwifery text of the time, using the question-answer catechistic format, informed readers that it was a normal event beginning with menarche at 14 or 15, and known as the monthlies, ordinaries, flowers or menses. McClive shows that the importance of the text is diagnostic, enabling recognition of the cause of any blood breaking the body's boundaries, but she also cautions that all blood loss was considered to be connected with menstruation.[57] This is evidence of the continuing dominance of Classical Greek and Roman ideas in Western thought about women's surplus blood being evacuated, and which carried through in medical thought until the 18th century.

During the 17th century in England, attitudes to menarche and menstruation were influenced by more complex beliefs about blood, life and death arising from Christian teachings and articulated by men in a culture of male dominance, according to historian Patricia Crawford.[58] Cause and effect are argued in perceptions of women's physiological inferiority situating them in positions of social inferiority. Crawford discusses the impact of the printing press in the 16th century, allowing the literate access to medical knowledge of menstruation, previously the realm of male medical

56   B.J. Sokol, '"Tilted lees", dragons, haemony, menarche, spirit, and matter in Comus', *The Review of English Studies*, vol. 41, no. 163, 1990, pp. 309, 310, 311, 312, 324. See also Dean-Jones (2001), p. 228.

57   Cathy McClive, 'Menstrual knowledge and medical practice in early modern France c. 1555–1761', in *Menstruation: a Cultural History*, Andrew Shail and Gillian Howie (eds), Palgrave Macmillan, Basingstoke, 2005, p. 76.

58   Patricia Crawford, 'Attitudes to menstruation in seventeenth-century England', *Past and Present*, vol. 91, no. 1, 1981, p. 47–48.

practitioners, together with other forms of knowledge on the same topic, and using language as a key indicator to perceptions not necessarily held by women themselves.[59] Two dominant thoughts about the purpose of menarche and menstruation were kept alive. One, the Aristotelian model of purification through evacuation led to naming menstruation 'purgation'. The cause of the menarcheal or menstrual event was believed to be fermentation of the blood, which medical practitioners described as being similar in process to fermentation of wine or malt liquor in which scum, called flowers, is forced to the surface. The menstrual imitative with a characteristic odour and associated idea of impurity became known as 'flowers', although some believed the term entered common use as anticipation of a young woman's later bearing of fruit. In this naming, the conceptual dichotomy is clear and Crawford observes that by the 18th century, questions were being raised about the fermentation-purification theory.

The second idea about menarche and menstruation in 17th-century England also shows the influence of Aristotle. The female body was still believed to be an inferior version of the male, lacking the ability to utilise the blood concocted from food. According to Crawford, the medical practitioner Galen, in second-century Rome, believed menstruation to be a plethora of unused blood-substance that, given suitable circumstances, might have nourished a foetus or been converted to lactation. However, by 1707, political and medical writer James Drake was arguing against menstruation being the emission of a plethora. There was little shift in thought about late menarche in the 1600s, both in England and France, where it was given disease status (named greensickness), and associated with the same symptoms as it had in Classical Greece. The cure depended on how the medical practitioner understood menstruation, and might include blood-letting from the foot – not the arm, as that would not draw blood to the uterus or womb. Another recognised reason for an absence of menarche in young girls was over-exercise, thought to leave no surplus blood to be excreted, as Soranus had described in the early second century, with the same advice to change customary activities offered.[60]

Crawford found traces of women's voices living on in historical documents of the time, a rare presence. Certain facts are evident: the expectation of menstruation every four weeks; the aura of privacy and sometimes secrecy maintained by women toward menstruation; a dislike and avoidance

---

59 Crawford (1981), pp. 48–49.
60 Crawford (1981), pp. 50–51, 53–54. See also Soranus, *Gynaecology*, trans. Temkin (1991), p. 133.

of physical examination by 'groping doctors'; a resistance to medical practitioners' bloodletting for any absence of menstruation; and embarrassment over unexpected menarche or menstruation. In the main, women preferred to discuss concerns and cures among themselves or with midwives. It would be interesting to know if the women resisted blood-letting because they experienced a feeling of being less well as a consequence, in contrast with the medical belief in the treatment's efficacy. It appears that women viewed menstruation within the context of their reproductive potential and there is no reason to suppose the young menarcheal girl differed. There was no particular recognition of the rite of passage, according to Crawford, although the hiatus provided by maidenhood might well be considered a liminal stage of life. Once fully adult through marriage and childbirth, menstruation became a normal part of life for 17th-century women. In contrast with this, men perceived an ambiguity of power and weakness in women, which allowed them to define women's inferior place in society through menarche and menstruation.[61]

For historical demographers following trends in population studies, it not only indicates the age of marriage for girls but allows change to be followed in a wider context of famine, disease, warfare, attitudes, and values influenced by social movements such as acceptance of religious belief systems. For social historians the age of menarche helps explain socio-sexual conventions and relationships within a marriage framework. Medical practitioners may read it as indicative of a biological process with attendant risk. The curious reader will compare what is represented in the past with the known, and very different, present. Menarche at 13 we can understand. Marriage, under social duress, at 14 may seem premature unless we recognise it as a form of controlling sexual activity relative to particular cultures such as Classical Greek. The age of menarche continues to be a salient point in any society. The historian, Peter Laslett, associates rigorous social control with menarche, arguing that no community anywhere at any time, regardless of resources, can allow girls to reproduce at will. He suggests that the age of menarche, given as about 14 in medieval and early modern times, increased toward the 19th century.[62] This is borne out in studies of 827 women by Dr Nicolai Edvard Ravn in Denmark in 1848, providing evidence that the average menarcheal age was 15 years and 8½ months. Ravn observed the differences in social classes between girls who were from

---

61   Crawford (1981), pp. 67, 68, 69, 70, 71, 72.
62   Peter Laslett, 'Age of menarche in Europe since the eighteenth century', *Journal of Interdisciplinary History*, vol. 2, no. 2, 1971, p. 221, 223.

urban and rural communities. The earlier menarche of upper-class urban girls was due, he believed, to the refinement and stimulation of education and nutrition. In the rural sector the daughter of a non-farmer, classified as clergyman or teacher for example, had a slightly earlier menarche than her urban counterpart, for possibly the same reasons with the added benefits of country life.[63] Scholars in the field have been inclined to argue over variations in menarcheal ages. Social scientist Vern L. Bullough is critical of the claims of earlier menarche in Western Europe made by child health researcher J. M. Tanner, who asserted a difference of some four months per decade between 1830 and 1960. Not unreasonably, Bullough comments that the variants of genetics, diet, and skeletal maturation make it difficult to pinpoint a historically stable age of menarche.[64] Another aspect of the debate is given by historical demographer J.B. Post, who believes Tanner's menarche statistics to be the best available in the West for the 19th and 20th centuries, but cautions that the same method that provided evidence of the decline referred to above would have placed menarche in the mid-20s c.1650. Post argues that a suggested retardation of menarche, beginning in Europe about 1500, is not borne out in a 15th-century gynaecological text that refers to menarche at twelve, 'purgations from the tyme of .xij'.[65] He contends greater accuracy regarding age of menarche exists in writings intended for textbook use by medical practitioners informed by patients.[66]

In 18th-century England, male midwives were responsible for an increased focus on menarche and menstruation. The rise of the male midwife, according to medical historian Irvine Loudon, advanced the knowledge, if not the care, of women. However, it is the knowledge that we are concerned with here. As for the male midwives: by and large they had served an apprenticeship to barber-surgeons and then hung up their boards. Some took advantage of the new courses offered by the University of Edinburgh and in London, the latter being the learning place of William Smellie, notable for his manoeuvre used in breech (feet-first) deliveries. By the end of the 18th century the position of the male midwife was well

---

63 E. Manniche, 'Age at menarche: Nicolai Edvard Ravn's data on 3385 women in mid-19th century Denmark', *Annals of Human Biology*, vol. 10, no. 1, 1983, pp. 79–81.
64 Vern L. Bullough, 'Age at menarche: a misunderstanding', *Science*, vol. 213, no. 4505, 1981, pp. 365–366. See also letters by J. M. Tanner and Peter T. Ellison, 'Menarcheal age', *Science*, vol. 214, no. 4521, 1981, p. 604.
65 The 'j' is the elongated 'i' used in manuscripts of the time: 'xij' is 12.
66 J.B. Post, 'Ages at menarche and menopause: some medieval authorities, *Population Studies*, vol. 25, no. 1, 1971, pp. 83, 87. The citation is from MS Corpus Christi College 69, 119a, p. 87.

established.[67] Historian Alexandra Lord observes that the lines between male midwives and physicians blurred, making differentiation between their professional categories difficult. At the time, menstruation in Britain was widely considered to cause and define weakness in the bodies of women. Lord argues that it was an issue that drew medical theorists' attention and presented the male midwife with an opportunity to move beyond childbirth to treat women who had problems with menstruation, or catamenia as it was known, and hence improve their general health. Rather than disregard the knowledge accrued from the ancients and medievalists, they chose to build upon it or disprove it. Three theories were discarded: that menstruation was a response to lunar forces, that it was a fermentation of the blood, and that it was an excretion of bodily excess.[68]

Menarche was a focus of close attention by these practitioners. Climatic effect was argued to influence age of onset; consequently girls living in warm to tropical climates had an earlier menarche than those living in temperate weather conditions. Lord argues an English aversion to premature menarche because transformation of the child's body to pubescent excess was associated with perceptions of early sexuality and immorality, in an unwelcome process with connotations of uncleanliness. In contrast, girls who experienced a late menarche were spared the implicit suggestions of sexuality and immorality and were able to adopt the socially approved role of being 'delicate'. Situations of menarcheal difficulty, diagnosed by scant bleeding, were almost certainly worsened by a diagnosis that correlated blood loss and narrowed uterine blood vessels. Echoes of the Hippocratics were present in the wide belief that childbirth was the cure. There may have been no recommended defloration by marriage, as the Hippocratics advised, but there was intervention by the practitioner, supposedly to release trapped excess blood thought to be potentially toxic. This invasion of the virginal body was not without medical critique, some arguing that a late menarche was natural for certain girls. Parents, particularly those of the upper class, also resisted the intervention, believing hymenal presence in their daughters was a necessary indication of

---

67   Irvine S. Loudon, 'Childbirth', in *Companion Encyclopedia of the History of Medicine, Vol. 2*, (1993), W.F. Bynum and Roy Porter (eds), Routledge, London 1997, pp. 1051–1053. Training, certification and practice of English midwives did not come under the Midwives Act until 1902. Until that time traditional practice was widely carried out and some practice by trained nurses. See Margaret Myles, *Textbook for Midwives*, Churchill Livingstone, Edinburgh 1975, p. xxiv.

68   Alexandra Lord, "The Great Arcana of the Deity' menstruation and menstrual disorders in eighteenth-century British medical thought', *Bulletin of the History of Medicine*, vol. 73, no. 1, 1999, pp. 39, 44.

virginity. The outcome of this focus on menarche and menstruation was a growing perception of fragility in the young female body and a continuing uncertainty about the cause and effect of menarche and menstruation among the practitioners.[69]

In 1896 W. E. Fothergill wrote his *Manual of Midwifery* as a teaching text intended for the University of Edinburgh, with greater theoretical knowledge necessitating two revisions before 1903. Fothergill makes the observation that menarche ushers in 'a periodic disturbance marked by a discharge of blood from the mucous membrane of the uterus, mixed with cellular detritus and mucus from the whole of the genital tract', indicating that dissection of uteri at various parts of the cycle had been undertaken with a resultant change in understanding of process. However, the most significant comment made by Fothergill links ovulation to menstruation:

Periodic sanguineous discharge occurs only in homo and some of the higher apes, whereas ovulation is a process essential to sexual reproduction throughout the organic world. The periodic 'rut' or 'heat' of many animals – a time of pelvic congestion, mucous discharge, and sexual appetite – is closely related with the ripening of ova. The relation of menstruation to ovulation is less clear.[70]

The following year J. K. Watson's *A Complete Handbook of Midwifery* was published, giving further evidence of theoretical knowledge built on the foundation of Aristotle. We read of pre-menarcheal development of 'the throat and chest' as one of the 'outward signs combined with certain internal changes we shall now discuss under the terms ovulation and menstruation' but:

We do not yet know the precise relation which ovulation bears to menstruation. Some say the two are independent. Ovulation has been said to commence before menstruation. Ovisacs may, it has been averred, ripen and burst in childhood. A case has been recorded where a woman was delivered of a child before menstruation had set in, which would form an argument for their independence ... menstruation usually commences between fourteen and fifteen, but it occurs earlier in warm climates, and also among the richer classes of society.[71]

---

69   Lord (1999), pp. 46, 49–51, 60.
70   W. E. Fothergill, *Manual of midwifery for the use of Students and Practitioners*, William F. Clay, Edinburgh 1903, p. 16.
71   J. K. Watson, *A Complete Handbook of Midwifery for Midwives and Nurses*, The Scientific Press Limited, London, 1904, pp. 21–23, 26.

How did this knowledge come about and what was its implication for menarcheal girls? To begin, an association between ovarian function and menstruation was first hypothesised by John B. Daveridge in 1793. His theory remained of little interest to medical knowledge before 1860.[72] Nevertheless, in 1840, a zoologist, Felix A. Pouchet, had made a connection between animals and humans, asserting that ovulation occurred during oestrus, and that human menstruation and animal oestrus, both observable, corresponded.[73] Further studies on Macacus Rhesus monkeys were taken up by Cambridge embryologist Walter Heape, who suggested menstruation was a degenerative process in preparation for oestrus.[74] In 1874 obstetrician John Williams presented post-mortem findings on menstruating women to the Royal Society of London and in 1875 presented further findings on the link between ovulation and menstruation.[75] Further to this, the medical historian Helen Blackman provides us with the context in which the work was carried out. It was a time of concern about British supremacy, and of alarm regarding eugenics in relation to changes in women's social roles.[76] Embryologist George Corner argues that from the 1890s agriculturalists, anthropologists, embryologists and obstetricians searched for answers to physiological problems that challenged the skills of gynaecologists, lacking in both understanding of the menstrual cycle and a sound basis of biological knowledge.[77] Corner maintains, incorrectly, that in Britain the research subjects were animals.[78] Meantime in Germany Robert Schroeder and Robert Meyer identified the general pattern of women's cycles. Working with human material, they found that ovulation occurred mid-cycle and that menstruation did not parallel animal oestrus but followed the transformation of ovum to corpus luteum.[79] It would be some years before work on higher primates revealed menstruation can occur without ovulation,

72   George W. Corner, 'Our knowledge of the menstrual cycle, 1910–1950', *The Lancet*, 28 April 1951, p. 919. This was the fourth annual Addison Lecture given at Guy's Hospital, London, 13 July 1950.

73   Helen Blackman, 'Embryological and agricultural constructions of the menstrual cycle, 1890–1910, in *Menstruation: a Cultural History*, Andrew Shail and Gillian Howie (eds), Palgrave Macmillan, Basingstoke, 2005, p. 118.

74   Corner (1951), pp. 920–921.

75   Graily Hewitt, *The Pathology, Diagnosis, and Treatment of the Diseases of Women*, fourth edition, Longmans, Green, and Company, London, 1882, pp. 15–16, 19.

76   Blackman (2005), p. 118.

77   Corner (1951), p. 919.

78   Apart from Williams, Hewitt, as Professor of Midwifery and Diseases of Women at the University Hospital, London, documents immediate post-mortems on menstruating women. See Hewitt (1882), pp. 16–17.

79   Corner (1951), pp. 919–920.

as it does at menarche and for some time thereafter. The corpus luteum does indeed cause change to the endometrium, but menstrual bleeding is not because of this change but rather because the change ceases.[80] The practical outcome of this knowledge was recognition of the time ovulation occurs in women. That knowledge was the basis for further studies in fertility control and the place of ovarian hormones in the cycle. Continuing research led to reproductive technology as we know it today. Corner commented in 1951 that the functional significance of menstruation remained unknown. The question as to why it was specific in such a developed form to only certain female primates and humans remained unanswered.[81] Recently, veterinary scientist Colin Finn argued menstruation to be a relic of the prehistoric Müllerian duct in primitive vertebrates, which permitted internal fertilisation and survival of the embryo on land.[82] Eventual merging together of the duct and embryo meant changes to the duct, evolving from embryonic demand for food and protection which resulted in its deep implantation. The uterine response was endometrial changes in anticipation of this invasion. When this failed to occur, the endometrium disintegrated in blood as menstruation.[83] Against this we may read a description of menstruation by William Ledger from a recent edition of Dewhursts's highly respected textbook on obstetrics and gynaecology:

> Menstruation refers to the shedding of the superficial layers of the endometrium, with subsequent repair in preparation for regrowth from the basal layer. Menstruation is initiated by a fall in circulating concentration of progesterone that follows luteal regression – failure of 'rescue' of the corpus luteum by an implanted early pregnancy. Luteal progesterone synthesis is dependent on luteinising hormone from the pituitary gland. During luteolysis, progesterone secretion falls despite maintained serum concentrations of luteinising hormone, since the

---

80   Corner (1951), p. 921.
81   Corner (1951), p. 922.
82   The Müllerian duct, named after German scientist Johannes Peter Müller (1801–1858), referred to an embryonic paired duct system from which the epithelial lining of the female reproductive organs – uterine tube, uterus and vaginal vault – developed. The male gonadal development degenerated under the influence of the duct system. See Mark Hill, 'Müllerian duct', http://www.embryology.med.unsw.edu.au/notes/index/m.htm.
83   Colin A. Finn, 'Why do women menstruate? Historical and evolutionary view', *European Journal of Obstetrics and Gynaecology and Reproductive Biology*, vol. 70, nos. 3–8, 1996, pp. 4, 7.

corpus luteum becomes less sensitive to gonotrophic support and becomes increasingly unable to maintain production of progesterone.

In the immediate pre-menstrual phase, progesterone withdrawal activates a complex series of intrauterine signals which include expression of chemotactic [response to chemical] factors, which draw leucocytes [white blood cells] into the uterus, and expression of ... other compounds that act on the uterine vessels and smooth muscles. The 'invasion' of leucocytes and subsequent expression of inflammatory mediators has led to menstruation being likened to an inflammatory event. Increased production of one type of prostaglandin produces contraction of the middle uterine layer and constriction of the blood vessels seen at menstruation, while another variation of prostaglandin increases pain and swelling, and dilates the blood vessels, inducing another key inflammatory and chemotactic mediator. Pronounced vasoconstriction in turn leads to localised tissue hypoxia [lack of oxygen] increasing release of inflammatory mediators. The end result of this cascade of events is constriction of the spiral arterioles [small arteries] with contraction of the uterine muscles, leading to expulsion of the shed tissue.[84]

Another aspect is Ledger's likening of menstruation to an inflammatory event. This builds on the theory of it being an ovarian event. Moreover, Ledger's account is not incompatible with Finn's hypothesis of the functional significance of menstruation. We can see the presence of blood, the main symbol of the healthy adult woman, has no association with the Classical or ancient belief in menstruation being a bodily excess or purgation. Clearly, this theory of menstruation has been influenced by the knowledge and understanding of endocrinology following the work of researchers a century ago. Has it altered any concepts about menarche? D. Keith Edmonds in Dewhurst's textbook suggests an expansion in thought about the psycho-logical development of the menarcheal girl, arguing a greater awareness of self-identity. The familiar secondary sex characteristics, breast development and axillary and pubic hair, are noted. The Aristotelian influence in evidence in Watson's 'throat and chest development' has lost credence. Additional

---

84   William L. Ledger, 'The Menstrual Cycle', in *Dewhurst's Textbook of Obstetrics and Gynaecology*, seventh edition, D. Keith Edmonds and John Dewhurst (eds), Wiley-Blackwell, Oxford, 2007, p. 354. Minor editing for non-medical understanding has been made.

knowledge includes more attention to the growth spurt, which may be as much as eight centimetres in one year, occurring about two years before menarche. This is arrested by the production of oestrogen, which closes the growth points of the long bones so that final height is reached around 14 to 15 years. The onset of menarche is influenced by genetics and by hormones. A recently advanced theory, concerning transforming growth factors, includes that of the epidermis which links to an increase in body fat. There is also an association with external factors such as socio-economic background, nutrition and dietary habits and psychological profile, which might include anorexia nervosa or obesity. Early menstrual cycles are thought to remain non-ovulatory, possibly even for as much as 5–8 years, before regularity of cycle is established, and potential heavy blood loss is due to production of progesterone without ovulation.[85] There is no mention of menarcheal girls being either 'delicate' or in a 'perilous' state of their lives.

Conclusion

The transition from child to woman, symbolised by menarche, has throughout history been a focus of the evolving thoughts, beliefs and actions of male medical practitioners, concerned to understand, to define and often also to control the menarcheal body. The meanings attributed to menstrual blood were a key feature of this control. In Classical Greek society menarche was constructed as commencement of the vital overflow of unused nourishment, made possible by widened blood vessels. Control was practised by the construction of a social age of onset, necessitating male intervention to correcting the health hazards of failure to bleed. The role of women in this control is uncertain, but the association in Classical Rome between menarche, dowry and marriage would suggest the practice had some support by women.

The onset of menarche in Ancient Chinese thought related to the function of other organs and served as a guide to the health of a young girl. In the Imperial Court in medieval China, menarche was associated with growing sexual desire, and early marriage followed among upper-class girls. Social control was apparent in the influence of a court physician, Chu Cheng, who prohibited sexual knowledge and marriage for a decade after menarche. In ancient India, Ayurvedic thought did not include any recommended form of social control relating to girls at menarche. In writings by men, menarche

---

85   D. Keith Edmonds, 'Gynaecological disorders of childhood and adolescence', in
      Dewhurst's Textbook of Obstetrics and Gynaecology (2007), p. 366.

was constructed symbolically as the meeting of two principles, water and fire, and the male perspective was evident in the fabled interpretation of the demonic child-killer as an example of the fate awaiting girls who reach 16 without menstruating.

Christian religious and social elite in late medieval England constructed an ideal of nubile perfection, symbolised by the Virgin Mary, as a control of the body of the young menarcheal girl. This occurred at a time when canonical law defined the age of consent as 12, and indicates cooperation between the Church and girls and young women, which resulted in the cult of virgin martyrdom, with its long-lasting influence on the English construction of the ideal woman. An alternative construction of menarche is seen in the work of Milton, where it is depicted as the time of a young woman's recognition of her sexual power through virgin non-acquiescence, and indicates an awareness of growing agency among young women. This was furthered in women's documented dislike of, and resistance to, medical examinations and interventions based on the Aristotelian influence of purification through evacuation. Classical Greek thought continued to influence medical and social ideas about women's bodies as inferior until the 18th century, as did the persistent medical construct of late-onset menarche as sickness.

From the late 19th century a widening scientific knowledge and understanding of women's blood, menarche and menstruation continued to accumulate. Western medical thought remained dominant in shaping social attitudes and policies that influenced the ways in which young women would live. Today, remnants of older beliefs that have survived are heard in the testimony of some of the interviewees. The reader might ask where the ideas originated. This overview is intended to provide answers.

Chapter 2

THE SHOCKED AND THE SANGUINE

I saw my blood ... what happened to me?[1]

When we think back to our menarche we have all got stories to tell. Memories of time and place, the moment of disbelief at what we saw, the getting used to our own blood and struggling for ways to contain it, the comfort of mothers and close friends, and the stories we were told about what to do and what not to do all contributed to what was an entirely new part of life. As happy as we may have been to confide in close friends and to be confided in, our menarche remained a private concern. Thirty years ago some interest in the social element of menstruation increased in Western societies, but there was little research on the actual meaning of menarche to girls, or of how the experience fitted their expectations.[2] This remains the case in Australia today. Although menarche signifies the change from early puberty to maturation by the onset of bleeding, the beginning of a physiological function specific to women, there are differences among individuals, including the age of onset, quantity and duration of blood loss, the presence or absence of accompanying discomfort, and the emotional acceptance or resistance to physical change. In addition to these aspects, I was interested in finding if there was any cultural influence in the ways in which young girls thought about menarche, and also if practices associated with it were intended as methods of control over the newly menstruating body.

My research introduced me to women from many cultures. With one exception, all had experienced menarche in countries outside Australia, and many before the advent of electronic media. Their testimony indicates

---

1   Meletta, 13 years old at menarche, Egypt, year unknown.
2   Virginia L. Ernster, 'Expectations about menstruation among pre-menarcheal girls', *Medical Anthropology Newsletter*, vol. 8, no. 4, 1977, p. 17.

that, apart from the confusion many had felt, the major understanding of menarche was not constructed by the event itself but by knowledge, cultural attitudes and values imparted by those they informed. This was where meaning was made, and here it might be opportune to explain what I mean by culture. The term has many interpretations, depending on where you might be coming from theoretically, but here I mean: constantly evolving systems of human actions and thought specific to a group of people. Within these systems meanings are embedded in language and social process. Cultural analyst William Sewell proposes two well-defined meanings. One, as a theoretical category of social life constructed from the many facets of human life and two, as a body of beliefs and practices shaped within a tangible and circumscribed world.[3] Decidedly ambiguous meanings continued to be attached to menstruation, while in many non-Western countries menarche and menstruation remained topics unfit for general discussion because they were considered 'dirty'.[4] Close family members, and that included sisters, frequently practised silence. Consequently for many girls menarche was a time of 'mixed messages', as a young girl tried to negotiate her way through a preview of life as an adult woman.

My interviewees experienced menarche between 1934 and 1969, and their memories are arranged according to the topic under discussion rather than according to culture, age or chronology, in the interests of identifying cultural similarities and differences in non-quantitative data interpretation. The focus is on four questions: what was their initial response to the moment of seeing blood external to the body's boundary? Whom did they tell? What was the immediate response of that person? What were the broader social responses to the event? It will be shown that the experience of menarche was influenced by prior knowledge of the event and the responses have been grouped accordingly. Some women, as girls, were ignorant or had failed to absorb an earlier explanation; two took an ostrich head-in-the-sand approach that if they ignored the bleeding it would disappear; others associated their blood with disease; some were traumatised by the experience; several had some prior information about menstruation. So there are elements of shock balanced with some sanguinity at what might be called an extra-ordinary happening. On reflection, the same response is not

---

3   William Sewell, Jr., 'The concept(s) of culture', in *Beyond the Cultural Turn: New Directions on the Study of Society and Culture*, Victoria E. Bonnell and Lynn Hunt (eds), University of California Press, Berkeley, 1999. p. 39.
4   K.P. Skandhan, Amita K. Pandya, Sumangala Skandhan, Yagnesh B.Mehta, 'Menarche: prior knowledge and experience', *Adolescence*, vol. 23, no. 89, 1988, p.151.

uncommon to loss of the first tooth, but there is some sort of mystique with menarche that is absent from other milestones in the passage to adulthood that I shall try to identify. In structuring this voyage of exploration I will be mindful of American women's studies academic Janet Lee and researcher in adult development and ageing Jennifer Sasser-Coen, who, in a discourse of the menarcheal experience, describe women's stories as an interweaving of historical and socio-cultural knowledge and individual development.[5]

Stories from the first group who were either ignorant, or who had failed to absorb information given because it lacked relevance to them at the time, reveal a grappling with the unexpected but with a certain pragmatism. Athene, Greek, remembered being 'at school and I felt something wet. I did not know what it was'.[6] Violetta, Filipina, also at school, recalled, 'my teacher told me to go to the blackboard to write my homework. Because I have my homework I stand right away and then my classmate behind me pulled my dress. I said why, what's the matter? "You have blood on your clothes". So I sit down and the teacher told me to go to the blackboard and I said "I don't know Sir". That's what I answered the teacher and then he was angry, wanted to smack me, but did not'.[7] In this experience classroom achievement was negated by the physiological disturbance that compelled immediate response, demonstrating the interviewee's awareness of social silence and invisibility of menstruation. It was night when Sri Lankan Daksha noticed blood and her confusion is clear, possibly enhanced by end-of-day tiredness, 'when I want to go to bed I saw. I told my mother, "Mummy, Mummy what is happening? There is blood"'.[8] Netri, Indian, 'wondered what it was. Surprise'.[9] The plight of a young girl, alone, is conveyed in the memory of Saha, Indian: 'I got up and I saw that my panties had some blood. I have no mother. I had no one really close to me where I could go'.[10] Cultural class-structures determine reliance on servants to inform, and be informed of, bodily processes, as two interviewees established. Jung, Korean, recalled 'I didn't know and when I got up in the morning my maid discovered it',[11] and Ria, Filipina, remembered 'I was at home and I told my maid.

---

5   Janet Lee and Jennifer Sasser-Coen, *Blood Stories: Menarche and the Politics of the Female Body in Contemporary U.S. Society*, Routledge, New York 1996, p. 38.
6   Athene, 13 years old, Greece c.1956.
7   Violetta, 14, Philippines 1938.
8   Daksha, 13, Sri Lanka 1947.
9   Netri, 14, India 1951.
10   Saha, 13, India c.1957.
11   Jung, 13, South Korea 1959.

I said there's something red, something going on in my ... you know?"[12] Corazon, Filipina, reveals certain knowledge by association but is affected nevertheless: 'I was about to start my first year high school when I had a period. I had no preparation at all. What I knew of periods came from my cousins who lived with us. Every month I saw them washing their undies when they have all this, you know? I'm surprised. I have mixed feelings, you know? I'm overwhelmed actually at that time'.[13] For some, the menarcheal experience was fleeting and insignificant. Indonesian Rara recalled 'a day only in the pants, you know? My grandmother, old woman, not tell anything but next day my grandma gave me medicine'[14] and for Wani, also Indonesian, menarche was a nameless exudation – 'when I first had it I told my mother'.[15]

Two women adopted the 'ostrich approach' of ignoring what they saw in the hope it would disappear. Marjorie, English, 'was going to a church social and I was wearing my confirmation dress which was white crepe. I went to the toilet in the church hall and I saw some blood. I thought if I ignored it, it would go away',[16] and Karuna, an Indian in Kenya, saw that 'I had a little stain I thought maybe it was simply for some reason and kept quiet'.[17] Several of the women immediately connected menarcheal bleeding to sickness, and although there was a shared association, their responses were varied. Meletta, Greek living in Egypt, recalled 'when I went to the toilet to pass the urine I saw my blood, on toilet paper, some blood, and I say "what happened to me?"'[18] Italian Maria 'was at home but I was scared. I was ... scared. I didn't know what it was. I thought I was very sick'[19] and Zosime, Greek living in Egypt, harked back to how 'I make one fight with my brother. He hit me in the back. It was the start. I tell nobody. I was, like, stupid, I couldn't understand anything'.[20] Alla, Ukrainian, remembered that 'it was May and at school. Pain in the stomach. I went to the hospital and there they explained'.[21] Ruth, Ugandan, 'woke up and felt wet so I went to the latrine. We didn't have toilets. It was an outside latrine and I checked myself and it was blood. I thought ... something's wrong'.[22] Sicilian Rosalia's

12   Ria, 13, Philippines 1967.
13   Corazon, 11, Philippines 1956.
14   Rara, 12, Indonesia 1951.
15   Wani, 13, Indonesia 1954.
16   Marjorie, 12, England 1956.
17   Karuna, Kenya, age and year of menarche unknown.
18   Meletta, 13, Egypt, year unknown.
19   Maria, 14, Italy 1957.
20   Zosime, 11, Egypt 1934.
21   Alla, 14, Ukraine, year unknown.
22   Ruth, 17, Uganda c.1974.

experience was doubly memorable because 'it was Christmas Eve and I was crying. I didn't know what's happened to me and I called Mum and she said "why are you crying? What's wrong?" and I said I can't tell you and then I told her'.[23] Gloria, Filipina, was 'playing with the kids and then, something. I run. I run. I told my auntie there's something wrong with me. I'm sore. I'm bleeding. Look at it'.[24] Chinese-Vietnamese Bao recalled 'I not see nothing. My neighbour saw me [and asked] "when you got the pain of blood?" I said what's wrong with me?'[25]

The initial awareness of bleeding had caused considerable fear and made menarche a traumatic discovery for some of the women. There seems little doubt about the effect of the menarcheal discovery, although psychologists Diane Ruble and Jeanne Brooks-Gunn, in their examination of girls' reactions to menarche 30 years ago, asserted the experience was a negative reaction to disruption, particularly in girls who were unprepared in both timing and knowledge, rather than one of trauma.[26] Nevertheless, Italian Loretta remembers with some clarity, 'we had a vegetable garden and we watched these plants with cotton, and I sat like this, and my sister look at me, she say in Italian, "ooh, you have a period" because there was blood. I was crying, you know, because it was a shock'.[27] Chilean Melena returns to childish vernacular although, as her English lacked fluency, it may not be the terminology she uses: 'I felt something. I thought it may be wee-wee. I went to the toilet, saw, and cried, you know?'[28] Kateryna, Ukrainean, experienced shock at the unexpected: 'I was in the train in Ukraine. I saw blood. I was frightened'.[29] Italian Alcina 'was scared but I will tell to nobody when I have my period'.[30] Keshini, Sri Lankan, felt anxiety at her mother's reaction to the news of her menarche: 'I had my period at night but my mother saw it in the morning and she kept me inside. I didn't know anything but I felt a bit scared all of a sudden'.[31] Egyptian-born Jewish Yanuva's recollection conveyed the distress of the time: 'I'd been to the bathroom and I saw blood and I freaked. I came running down the stairs and yelled at the top of my

23   Rosalia, 13, Italy 1950.
24   Gloria, 13, Philippines 1959.
25   Bao, 12, Vietnam 1968.
26   Diane Ruble and Jeanne Brooks-Gunn, 'The experience of menarche', *Child Development*, vol. 53, no. 6, 1982, p. 1565.
27   Loretta, 10, Italy 1947.
28   Melena, 14, Chile, year unknown.
29   Kateryna, 15, Ukraine 1952.
30   Alcina, 15, Italy 1947.
31   Keshini, 12, Sri Lanka 1969.

voice to my parents who were somewhere in the corner, "Mummy, Mummy, there's blood. There's blood in the toilet".[32]

In a study of women's recollections, psychologists Sharon Golub and Joan Catalano argue that the significance of menarche as a life event enables the later, detailed recall of the circumstances.[33] For example, Virisila, Fijian, remembered 'the day was a Tuesday, and hurricane season, and we had been weeding in the rain. We all came in into our dormitories and I was wet. I went into the shower, turned on my shower, and I remember taking off my panty. It was called bloomers then, you know? I remember the colour was lemon with elastic at the (indicates waist and leg) and I looked at the stain and I remember feeling ooh my god, you know. I said ooh my god. I freaked out. I really freaked out and I came out with it without realising. I just ran out. I had nothing on and there were senior girls in the dormitory, like there were ten girls in there, but we had senior girls and I was one of the most juniors'.[34] The theme of shock was reported by others. Chilean Ramona remembered 'when I saw my first stain of blood I was shocked. I knew it, but I was shocked because I didn't know where the blood was coming from'.[35] Aleli, Filipina, echoed Ramona. 'When I first saw it I was really shocked. I was feeling "oh, my God". I couldn't tell anyone'.[36] Fear of the unknown, of being scared, was a widely shared response. Korean Sun recalled 'I just nervous and scared'.[37] Lola, Chilean, thought back, 'I was a little bit scared in the way it was coming because I was playing basketball at that moment'.[38] Nila, Sri Lankan, recounted that 'I knew this would happen to you and you were supposed to tell your parents or lady. I did. I felt scared'.[39] Chinese-Vietnamese Tu's memory was of being 'really scared and I go to school and I don't know how to use so I go to toilet all the time. After, I go home because all wet'.[40]

Previous knowledge combined with a certain emotional maturity reduced concern about menarche. In their study on the significance of subjective and objective timing for menarche, the psychologists Jill Rierdan and Elissa Koff

---

32   Yanuva, 10, Egypt 1957.
33   Sharon Golub and Joan Catalano, 'Recollections of menarche and women's subsequent experiences with menstruation', *Women and Health*, vol. 8, no. 1, 1983, pp. 58–59.
34   Verisila, 11, Fiji 1964.
35   Ramona, 15, Chile 1964.
36   Aleli, 10, Philippines 1959.
37   Sun, 13, South Korea 1962.
38   Lola, 17, Chile 1967.
39   Nila, 13, Sri Lanka 1964.
40   Tu, 14, Vietnam 1963.

found that, by early adolescence, children have formulated a social clock regarding life events that registers a sense of progress in comparison with peers. Girls who sense themselves to be either on time or late at menarche have a more favourable experience than the girl who perceives herself as too early, thus deviant, within her peer group. The girl who considers herself late is reincorporated among her peers by her menarche, no longer the deviant by absence, and is reassured of normality.[41] For instance, Cecile, Ugandan, recalled 'it happened at night, but, because I was a bit late having my period I knew what it was and also I'd seen some girls at school'.[42] Armenian Seda explained, 'I go to the toilet and explore. No, check for it, you know. Then I forgot about it but when it came I am in readiness'.[43] Fijian Levani recalled 'I went home and realised that, yes, it is a period, even though I didn't quite know what it was going to be like'.[44] Lee, Singapore Chinese, was pragmatic: 'I was watching television and I knew something's happening, you know? Not comfortable. Went to check, and I get a pad out, just use it, and went back to watch television. That's it'.[45] Nadia, Egyptian-born Lebanese, remembered, 'I said you were talking about that period and I saw blood in my undies. Is that a period?'[46] Qing, Hong Kong Chinese, recollected that 'when I first saw the stain of blood I was not shocked because I have the prior knowledge. My initial feeling is a combination of fear and happiness'.[47] Chilean Beatriz asked 'what? My turn now? I have to copy my sister. I know how to be like my sister but my sister was very scared about it and I am not going to be'.[48] Erlinda, Filipina, 'was aware and I wasn't scared'.[49] Indian Hetal remembered 'when I'm in ninth class, age of fourteen years, there are spots. I am living with my auntie and uncle but I have the liberty to have a cloth and put it on'.[50] Indonesian Nirmala said 'when it came I told my mum that there's this bleeding'.[51] Greek Elena was prepared: 'I feel something wet before telling the girls, my friends. I know a bit from the friends and I'm ready. No fright'.[52]

---

41   Jill Rierdan and Elissa Koff, 'Timing of menarche and initial menstrual experience', *Journal of Youth and Adolescence*, vol. 14, no. 3, 1985, pp. 238–242.
42   Cecile, 14, Uganda 1965.
43   Seda, 14, Armenia, year unknown.
44   Levani, 16, Fiji 1967.
45   Lee, 13, Singapore 1962.
46   Nadia, 11, Egypt 1950.
47   Qing, 12, Hong Kong 1962.
48   Beatriz, 12, Chile c.1960.
49   Erlinda, 12, Philippines 1964.
50   Hetal, 14, India c.1952.
51   Nirmala, 13, Indonesia 1964.
52   Elena, 14, Greece, year unknown.

With the exception of Violetta, the immediate discovery of menarche carried no socio-cultural overlay beyond fear of bleeding from an unknown cause, fear of which, according to physician Raymond Crawfurd, is universal.[53] The young girls simply saw blood as bodily matter and interpreted their finding according to their knowledge. Their stories support Lee and Sasser-Coen's assertion that there is no typical experience or response by girls to menarche, but one ultimately shaped by the cultural, socio-political and historical contexts in which the event takes place.[54] The experiences of the younger girls, Aleli, Loretta, Yunuva and Virisila at 10 and 11, support findings by Koff, Rierdan and Karen Sheingold that the younger the girl is at menarche, the less prepared she will be, and the more likely her interpretation of the experience is to involve shock and fear. They comment on aspects of memory over time, finding memory of subjective events to be less reliable than that for objective events, but that more harmful recollections of the subjective are minimised in recall.[55] In a later paper, David Pillemer and Elizabeth Rhinehart with Koff and Rierdan study so-called flashbulb memories of menarche, and find that the younger the girl, the greater the lack of understanding of the event in terms of both cause and effect. She is without any existing mental framework in which to place the experience. As a result her memories are vivid and episodic with future attitudes and behaviours informed by an elaborate memory of the event.[56] This is certainly exemplified by Loretta and Virisila's fragmented yet vivid memories of colour and place. Among the young girls who were informed about menstruation, factual details of menarche were of less significance.[57]

On becoming aware of the bleeding, most of the girls confided their experience to another woman. Years later the response is remembered, as Rhonda Andresen from Samoa, who was at boarding school in New Zealand at her menarche, recalls: 'I remember when I first got my period, I ran to the nuns. I had one I could go to who was a grandmotherly type

53 Raymond Crawfurd, 'Notes on the superstitions of menstruation, *The Lancet*, 18 December 1915, p. 1335.

54 Janet Lee and Jennifer Sasser-Coen, 'Memories of menarche: older women remember their first period', *Journal of Aging Studies*, vol. 10, no. 2, 1996, p. 64.

55 Elissa Koff, Jill Rierdan, Karen Sheingold, 'Memories of menarche: age, preparation, and prior knowledge as determinants of initial menstrual experience, *Journal of Youth and Adolescence*, vol. 11, no. 1, 1982, pp. 7–8.

56 David B. Pillemer, Elissa Koff, Elizabeth D. Rhinehart, Jill Rierdan, 'Flashbulb memories of menarche and adult menstrual distress, *Journal of Adolescence*, vol. 10, no. 2, 1987, p. 189.

57 Pilmer et al (1987), p. 196.

and was very, very kind'.[58] For most girls it is their mother who provides information and support at menarche, and this become a major theme in psychoanalytic texts.[59] Some women display an unresolved resentment when their mother's response is evoked over 50 years after the event. Lee and Sasser-Coen in their investigation of older American women's memories of menarche maintain that recollections, reconstructed in the present, reveal not just the event but later subjectivities and meanings attributed to the event, developed through the women's life experiences.[60] Maternal response influences how the meaning of menarche will be constructed, introducing social and cultural interpretations of menstruation that will be internalised by the young girl. For instance, Mary Suan from Manus Island reflects on the mother–daughter relationship as one 'never that close because some things just cannot be talked about'. Mary carried this tradition on into her own relationship with her daughter: 'anything personal like "I did my period" I would say "look, just go and ask your aunties", I can never talk to her because of my home background where it is forbidden'.[61] There were other reasons for silence as historian Joan Jacobs Brumberg found in her study on the development of what she calls the 'American hygiene imperative'. Among older Italian immigrants to the United States, mothers had rarely informed their daughters about menstruation or reproduction because of the cultural value placed on female virtue and purity.[62] At menarche, mothers' advice was both cautionary and associated with ideas of illness, as Italian Maria discovered when her mother 'warned me I would get it once a month. She said you'll get pains in your stomach and she said not to use cold water'.[63]

Brumberg found that within her oral history interviews, Jewish mothers also revealed lack of communication with their daughters.[64] Yanuva remembered being in Genoa, in transit from Egypt to Australia, and how 'my mother immediately took my sister and said "go for a walk and tell her all about it'. When we came back she said 'did you understand everything? Now

---

58 Rhonda Andresen, 'Hawai'i', in Debbie Hippolite Wright, Rosalind Meno Ram, Kathleen Fromm Ward (eds), *Narratives and Images of Pacific Island Women*, Women's Studies, Volume 44, The Edwin Mellen Press, Lewiston, NY, 2005, p. 123.

59 Ernster (1977), p. 23.

60 Lee and Sasser-Coen (1996), p. 84.

61 Mary Suan, 'More islands', in Wright et al (eds) (2005), p. 226.

62 Joan Jacobs Brumberg, '"Something happens to girls": menarche and the emergence of the modern American hygienic imperative', *Journal of the History of Sexuality*, vol. 4, no. 1, 1993, p.120.

63 Maria, 14, Italy 1957.

64 Brumberg, 'Something happens to girls' (1993), p. 120.

we don't talk about it'".[65] Lack of communication is also evident in the small secular ritual of face-slapping which is not peculiar to the Jewish tradition, being also associated with women in rural Turkey and Eastern Europe. It is a response by the mother on hearing of her daughter's menarche and in a mother's absence may be the prerogative of a female relative. Yanuva, confused and frightened by the menarcheal event, said 'I can't remember whether my sister slapped my face or told me that she ought to slap my face. I really can't remember … but I think she did slap it and told me that she got slapped when it happened to her'. Both the origin of, and reason for, this ritual are unclear. Yanuva was uncertain: 'I think it's probably to do with moving from one area of life to another … I really don't know'. Feminist Emma Goldman, who experienced her menarche in Russia in 1880, recalled the unexpectedness of her mother's slap, together with an explanation that Goldman found unacceptable: the slap represented 'protection against disgrace'.[66] Iliene Lainer, founder of New York's Centre for Autism, describes her shock and confusion, asking her mother what wrong she had done.[67] From the Museum of Menstruation and Women's Health, Caren Appel-Slingbaum argues face slapping to be a 'barbaric' custom, a *minhag* or old Jewish custom not in accordance with Jewish law despite being a tradition that had been passed through the generations.[68] Psychologist Ayse Uskal, interviewing women from Turkey, found the slap to be a cultural tradition lacking definitive meaning and varying in intent from bringing colour to the cheeks to being a tokenistic punishment for pride in having menstruated.[69] In every situation the custom appeared to cause additional distress for the menarcheal girl, particularly one who was very young, at a time when gentle reassurance was most needed.

Psychotherapist Jessica Gillooly, who works with mother and daughter relationships and teaches undergraduate psychology, asks students to write

65   Yanuva, 10, Egypt 1957.
66   Emma Goldman, cited in Delaney, Lupton and Toth (1988), p. 173.
67   Ilene Lainer, 'The Slap, 1972', in *My Little Red Book*, Rachel Kauder Nalebuff (ed.), Twelve, New York, 2009, p. 84.
68   Caren Appel-Slingbaum at the Museum of Menstruation and Women's Health, 'The tradition of slapping our daughters',, http:// www.mum.org/slap.htm, 2000.
69   Ayse K. Uskul, Women's menarche stories from a multicultural sample', *Social Science and Medicine*, vol. 59, no. 4, 2004, p. 676. Vera J. Milow, vice-president of educational affairs at Tampax Inc. was told the slap was to bring colour to the face, that it was symbolic of the threat the menarcheal girl's new sexuality brought to her mother and, similarly, it was a response to recognition of the girl as a sexual being. See Vera J. Milow, 'Menstrual education: past, present, and future', in *Menarche: The Transition from Girl to Woman*, Sharon Golub (ed.), Lexington Books, Lexington, 1983, p. 129.

their experiences of menarche. She finds girls accurately pick up on their mother's feelings about menstruation and are influenced accordingly.[70] Gillooly's findings are relevant to previous generations. For example Wani, Indonesian, recalled, 'I told my mother and I don't know why, she looked tense and she just said "ah, this is menstruation". I don't know why she was tense. I think she was an unhappy woman. My mother kept saying "you know being a woman is not a happy thing. It's a burden"'.[71] Later events showed Wani was not affected by her mother's attitude: 'I went on as usual. I learnt jiu-jitsu. I did other things, I was good at sports. Nothing happened'. Chilean Melena's experience was even less reassuring. 'She said "you know what? All women come to this" and folded toilet paper, "you start this, then you get back and you change". Very nasty. I wouldn't do that to my daughter. I cried and cried and my mum, this mother very rude. She upset, you know. No nice explanation'.[72] This contributed to Melena's developing attitude to menstruation as a physical hardship: 'why me? Why me? When my period was heavy and I'm going to school, I don't want to go to school'. In a study of how girls would recommend they be prepared for menstruation, Koff and Reardan found the maternal role to be complex. One of the many ambiguities that characterise the time of menarche is a girl's desire for emotional support and physical assistance from her mother, coupled with the need to achieve emotional distance from her. From the mother's viewpoint, her own emotional willingness or readiness to be involved with her daughter presents grounds for conflict, as we saw with Wani and Melena.[73] Consequently, an area is created for mother blaming, attributed to the unwanted negative messages given at menarche, which, according to psychologists Daryl Costos, Ruthie Ackerman and Lisa Paradis, are still embedded in today's American culture. Costos et al consider negative messages about menarche and menstruation to have been passed on and enforced by generations of women in Western cultures.[74] However it is reasonable to assert that mother blaming is not America-specific, but widely entrenched in cultures that promote silence between

---

70   Jessica B. Gillooly, 'Making menarche positive and powerful for both mother and daughter', *Women and Therapy*, vol. 27, no. 3, 2004.
71   Wani, 13, Indonesia 1954.
72   Melena, 14, Chile, year unknown.
73   Elissa Koff and Jill Rierdan, 'Preparing girls for menstruation: recommendations from adolescent girls', *Adolescence*, vol. 30, no. 120, 1995, p. 809.
74   Daryl Costos, Ruthie Ackerman, and Lisa Paradis, 'Recollections of menarche: communication between mother and daughter regarding menstruation' *Sex Roles*, vol. 46, nos 1/2, 2002, p.58.

mothers and daughters about matters related to menarche, menstruation and sexuality.

Women reported variations in their mother's responses to immediate needs. Meletta, Alexandrian-born Greek, recalled 'I tell Mum I need a towel that's special ... and she took me and showed me how to wash'.[75] Mothers who taught their daughters about menarche/menstruation also responded to their emotional and physical needs in ways remembered with affection, including through the agency of the daughter's friends. Violetta, Filipina, related how 'at recess time my classmate went to my house and told my mum that I was already having menstruation. So my mum gave her some clothes of mine and a napkin and we went to Home Economics and there I changed my clothes then I went to the class again'.[76] Emotional needs were met for Olena too: 'I show blood. Mama said that very good. You become woman ... you're normal ... no problems. Mama explained everything ... so I was not afraid'.[77] Fijian Virisila remembers with gratitude the understanding of a surrogate maternal figure at her boarding school. Her menarcheal needs were met when 'one of the senior girls was there. I remember saying her name and "I've got my period. What do I do?" And she said to me "don't worry, I'll show you", and she was about five, six years older than me'.[78] Absent mothers, who temporarily delegated others to act as maternal substitutes, resumed their position, ensuring old customs had not been forgotten. For Filipina Ria, the practice had added to her confusion, still apparent in the re-telling: 'my maid told me to do it. I'm panicking, you know, I saw blood in my undies ... you jump down from the stairs three or five steps. My mother came at night time. She told her about it. "Have you done it?" and she said "yeah, yeah". I can't remember what other things they said as I was still very young in those days'.[79] This cultural folkloric tradition was also recalled by Filipina Erlinda who had some prior knowledge of menarche. 'I told my mum. She said "that's what I'm telling you before, first blood of a woman". She said to jump from the stairs, three, one-two-three, and I jumped because she said it will take only three days for your menstruation to flow. She wet a towel and put it on my hair, on top of my head, to cool me down, she said because our blood is really hot'.[80] Trusted older sisters played

---

75   Meletta, 13, Egypt, year unknown.
76   Violetta, 14, Philippines 1938.
77   Olena, 11, Ukraine 1949.
78   Virisila, 11, Fiji 1964.
79   Ria, 13, Philippines 1955.
80   Erlinda, 12, Philippines 1964.

an important role in reassurance when menarche came early. Italian Neve remembered 'my sister say what is happening, "No worry. It's good because people who not have periods, they're sick"'.[81]

Some maternal responses involved designating person to who fulfill a particular role, a cultural practice that lead to a later public expression through ceremony. Sri Lankan Daksha reminisced about her mother's immediate reaction to her menarche. 'She said "you can wait today. You must go to your room." So I went to my room. We had to remove everything and when it's day time my mother bring the dhobi woman, they bring the clothes together. Seven days inside the house'.[82] Among other cultural groups menarche had associations with particular practices and caution with anyone other than close kin was necessary. A dimension of concern was added to Ugandan Cecile's experience. 'I was going to school. I was staying in another place with an auntie but I didn't tell her. I was told not to tell her, because she might do something, especially the first thing is very important'.[83]

Interestingly, in recent studies on the preparation for and experience of menarche, both Koff and Rierdan and Ruble and Brooke-Gunn found girls today place little emphasis on identity transformation to woman.[84] Three of the women I interviewed recalled feeling an identity transformation. Indian Hetal expressed it as 'already I am big. I feel proud'.[85] Lola said she was 'scared to see the blood but happy I was a woman'.[86] Erlinda, Filipina, 'had that feeling, you know, that I'm a real lady and I don't want to mix with girls anymore'.[87] The only woman who associated menarche with having the power of reproduction was Chinese Qing, who placed it in a cultural framework, 'if you don't have periods, suppose the secret is revealed, no man will take you'.[88] Women also recollected maternal responses associating menarche with sexuality. Greek Athene recalled how 'she tried to explain to me "you see, you are a woman now, be careful when you go out"'.[89] Retrospectively, Lebanese Maryam observed that 'parents want to protect their daughters, so when they know their daughters have their periods it becomes, you know, about falling pregnant. It's like she enters a danger zone in a way'.[90]

---

81   Neve, 11, Italy 1941.
82   Daksha, 13, Sri Lanka 1947.
83   Cecile, 14, Uganda 1965.
84   Koff and Rierdan, (1995), p. 808. See also Ruble and Brooks-Gunn (1982), p. 1565.
85   Hetal, 14, India c.1952.
86   Lola, 17, Chile 1967.
87   Erlinda, 12, Philippines 1964.
88   Qing, 12, Hong Kong 1962.
89   Athene, 13, Greece c.1956.
90   Maryam, 15, Lebanon 1942.

Young girls at menarche rarely self-identify as a sexual subject and may well find the information that they now have reproductive potential threatening.[91] There is little internalised connection between menarche and reproduction, and among the women interviewed there was ignorance and confusion about sexual matters at the time of menarche. English Marjorie thought back to 'when I started my periods I didn't know anything about sex. I thought if I stood next to a boy I could get pregnant so I used to cross the road if I saw a boy that I knew who might stop and talk to me. I'd just cross the road if I had my period. I didn't know how you conceived'.[92] Warnings given by mothers 'to be careful', were not understood because girls' lacked knowledge of conception. Fijian Virisila related that 'at home Mum didn't allow me to play as much. A lot of activities I used to do before my period she told me "don't do that … don't play with boys". I can't remember if I was interested in boys then'.[93] Cautionary warnings by mothers were particularly apparent in countries with a religious and socio-cultural emphasis on pre-marital chastity. In these patriarchal societies mothers acted as agents of control, and the warnings they gave were limited by the culturally censored framework of knowledge. Although the messages were clear, the practices that gave rise to them remain incomprehensible and create anxiety for the young girl, for instance', stay always away from a man or boy and especially when you've got your period. Be careful because you've become a big girl and you can get into trouble. Mum didn't discuss this', Sicilian Rosalia recalled.[94] The inference of menarche as a prelude to unknown sexual situations, placing the young girl in a defensive role, was further recalled by Chilean Ramona. 'No one knew in my family, just my mum and she cried with me saying "well, you have to be careful now" because of my virginity'.[95]

In her study of menarche as central to body politics, Janet Lee found a social response by parents in the immediate post-menarcheal months. Greater control over their daughters was exerted than at any other time and Chilean Beatriz recollected that 'the mum or the father started the rules. The rules were not to have a boyfriend, not to hide in a dark place or whatever. They have to look after themselves because they can get pregnant'.[96] Lee

---

91   Anne M. Teitelman, 'Adolescent girls' perspectives of family interactions related to menarche and sexual health', *Qualitative Health Research*, vol. 14, no. 9, 2004.

92   Marjorie, 12, England 1956.

93   Virisila, 11, Fiji 1964.

94   Rosalia, 13, Italy 1950.

95   Ramona, 15, Chile 1964.

96   Beatriz, 12, Chile c.1960; Janet Lee, 'Menarche and the (hetero) sexualization of the female body', *Gender and Society*, vol. 8, no. 3, 1994, p. 354.

argues that in heterosexual and patriarchal societies, menarche signals both sexual availability and reproductive potential and it is within this framework that the female body is placed, or places itself.[97] Levani, Fijian, remembered learning that 'you be careful with your relationship with men, boys. That was happening to me anyway because I was sixteen'.[98] Consequently, women's memories of menarche are constructed within competing discourses, one being the risk of potential pregnancy. Melena, Chilean, spoke of how 'the mother says "oh, I have to be more careful now. I have to control her". That's in our country for mothers'.[99] Nor does control stop with mothers. Lola, Chilean, remembered being puzzled about advice. 'I have to be a good girl, not around with boys because if I be with the boys I can be pregnant, but no explanation at all. I believe at that time we were very innocent people, not like now. I heard from my sister, my mother, my grandmother, that if you are with a boy you can be pregnant. I always believed that if I was holding hands I'd be pregnant, or if I was kissing him I'd be pregnant. I have to be careful with boys'.[100]

Two themes emerged from these stories. One is alienation, and Lee refers to 'alienated bodies', contending that women recalling menarche speak of themselves as passive objects of a bodily function over which they have no control. Menarche is an invader of the body, creating conflict with self, something to be struggled with, and regulated.[101] For instance, Indonesian Wani's 'when I first had it' recalled an experience made difficult by maternal attitude; English Marjorie's hopeful 'if I ignored it, it would go away'; Indian Karuna's attempt to explain 'maybe it was simply for some reason'; Italian Maria's fear of possible sickness, 'I didn't know what it was'; Ugandan Ruth's apprehensive 'I checked myself and it was blood'. None of the memories suggest any perception that menarche was part of the self, nor were the stories contextually framed within recollections of emergent awareness of sexuality as Lee theorises with her own interviews.

The second theme of dependence is generalised rather than age-dependent. Women who decided to be independent and cope alone at menarche contradicted the need for maternal help and support. Indian Sasha, at 13, without maternal or sororal support, had no option, but Italian Alcina was adamant, 'I will tell to nobody', and Greek Elena's 'no say to

---

97   Lee (1994), p. 344.
98   Levani, 16, Fiji 1967.
99   Melena, 14, Chile, year unknown; See also Lee (1994), p. 353.
100   Lola, 17, Chile 1967.
101   Lee (1994), pp. 349–350.

Mum. No say to anyone' are reflections on their individual belief that their bodies are their own. Both Elena and Alcina had older sisters so it may be hypothesised that both had witnessed family conflict and had made the conscious decision to avoid repetition beginning at their menarche. In his study on the psychological implications of menarche, Paul Trad discussed intra-family turbulence, triggered by divergent pubescent values and behaviours that contest established family rules. The effects produce change in the family structure, which Trad suggests may be an adaptive response, forcing the menarcheal girl to claim total independence from familial organisation by breaking away, physically and psychologically.[102] Trad's findings are borne out, albeit in a previous generation, 15-year-old Elena, the year after menarche, would 'take my boyfriend, go to Athens' and Alcina related how, within 12 months, 'I'd grown up and I go to live in Roma'.

Conclusion

Interviews indicated that individual responses to the first sighting of menarcheal blood are similar across cultures. Physical memories included the sensations of wetness and pain. Emotional responses commonly included shock, surprise, puzzlement, distress and fear of sickness. More positive responses included a mixture of fear and happiness, confidence and pride. Women without knowledge of menarche and menstruation, or those to whom such information appeared irrelevant at the time they received it, recalled being surprised but not shocked at onset; others had adopted the 'wait and see' approach due to ignorance of menstrual duration; yet others experienced fear that the blood indicated sickness, and remembered menarche as a traumatic event. Increased age at menarche and/or some knowledge of menstruation reduced concern over the discovery of bleeding. There was no cultural pattern apparent in any of these responses.

Women's recollections of communicating the onset of menarche to another person indicated mothers were the usual confidantes across cultures. In the immediate absence of mothers other women were informed: sisters, cousins, friends and maids, whose responses were sympathetic and in the main helpful, and a small number of women stressed their independence by concealing menarche from family. Attention was drawn to the mother–daughter relationship and the way in which menarche intensifies emotional responses. Deprivation of maternal support, help, interest and reassurance

---

102   Trad, Paul V., 'Menarche: a crossroad that previews developmental change', *Contemporary Family Therapy*, vol. 15, no. 3, 1993, pp. 231–232.

was recalled with some bitterness; conversely, maternal support given reduced the strangeness of the situation and promoted confidence. It strengthened the mother–daughter relationship and was remembered with gratitude.

The maternal figure determined cultural practices, commencing them when made aware of the situation. The most complex were found in Sri Lanka, where forms of ritual and seclusion followed the onset of menarche, and the simplest in the Filipina tradition of step-jumping. The small ritual act of face slapping was referred to by an interviewee as a practice of some Jewish mothers arising in Eastern European countries. Interviewees from countries where pre-marital chastity was emphasised recalled how their mothers' responses to their menarche linked the first period to growing sexual desire. Behavioural instructions included allusions to sexual practices, which were poorly understood by the majority of girls as they lacked knowledge of human reproduction. The girls' responses varied from ignorance and confusion, to rebellion, viewed briefly as two themes: body alienation and independence.

External to the interview data, studies indicate menarche is well remembered by women because of its significance in their lives, and that the memories are positively influenced by timely preparation for menstruation. This is evident in the interview data, which indicated little difference across cultures in the individual experiences and perceptions of menarche. Cultural practices introduced by the mother figure reflected cross-cultural differences, but with the shared intent of controlling the menarcheal body, which was framed as polluted, or sexualised. Consequently it is cultural-based traditions and activities such as these that influence the way in which women from diverse cultures construct their memories of menarche.

Chapter 3

BECOMING UNCLEAN

We are unclean when we've got the period.[1]

For many young girls the most disturbing feature of menarche is the involuntary secretion of blood from their bodies and the associated soiled clothing. Another aspect that came up early in the interview process was the concept of becoming unclean, in the sense of 'polluted'. As the interviews continued, women conveyed how their religion influenced their understanding of menarche and menstruation and expressed the thought that menarche introduced the presence of impurity or pollution to religious activities. Although these were older women, many emphasised that their beliefs were present in their cultures today. In this chapter I will argue that the religious belief systems observed by my interviewees – Judaism, Islam, Eastern and Western Orthodox Christian traditions, Hinduism and Buddhist thought – constructed the menstruating body of women as unclean, and that this influenced women's own constructions of the menstruating self. Throughout the chapter I will show ways in which the interviewees' religious belief systems governed practices relating to menstrual uncleanness. Moving beyond the interview data, I will explore the ways in which major shifts in thought regarding the pollutant qualities of the menstrual body came about in religious traditions.

Impurity and pollution were matters of major interest to anthropologist Mary Douglas, arising from her African fieldwork. Douglas develops the idea of dirt and contagion through two themes that the anthropologists Thomas Buckley and Alma Gottlieb noted are ideally suited to the topic of menstrual blood.[2] Douglas argues that ideas surrounding dirt are cultural

---

1   Bao, 12 years old at menarche, Vietnam 1968.
2   Thomas Buckley and Alma Gottlieb, 'A critical appraisal of theories of menstrual symbolism', in *Blood Magic: the Anthropology of Menstruation,* Thomas Buckley and Alma Gottlieb (eds), University of California Press, Berkeley, 1988, p. 26.

constructs, using as an example the guest given a cracked cup. Western social convention frames cracked drinking vessels as potentially harmful because dirt contains germs, so by transgressing custom the host endangers the guest by an action with the potential for contagion. In putting the cup aside, the idea of taboo is introduced, and from the simple everyday experience more complex theories are developed.

First is the concept of taboo, which Douglas argues is a way of maintaining a particular world-view of social organisation and stability. She links the study of taboo to belief systems, describing it as a coding function that sets up boundaries around potentially dangerous situations. Taboo works because of social compliance with belief and the authority of a leader, or leaders. Any contravention creates a threat that is potentially contagious to the entire community.

The second theme combines ambiguity and anomaly. Douglas argues that anything not fully understood, not able to be cognitively placed, causes concern, fear, and threat. Taboo provides protection by transferring the ambiguous to the bounded sacred.[3] Taboo also functions against cognitive unrest caused by the anomalous; Douglas refers to the Abominations of Leviticus and the pig, arguing that feet deviant from the cloven-footed domestic ruminants create the anomaly, hence uncleanness and dietary taboo. Although she uses the terms ambiguity and anomaly, she insists they are not synonymous. Ambiguity, for instance, is present in any situation or statement that may be interpreted in more than one way. If the ambiguous can be reduced to a single interpretation then the concern, fear, or threat is also reduced. Anomaly is the odd entity in any given group or series and causes the same concern, fear, and threat as ambiguity. However, the anomalous may be physically controlled by destruction of the cause, or by rules of avoidance, stressing oddity or difference as the converse of things approved. In all societies, 'matter out of place' – those anomalies and ambiguities considered unclean or dangerous, which William James describes as part of a system – must be set apart if order is to be preserved.[4]

A symbolic 'being set apart' was discussed by the first group of women interviewed, as part of articulating the concept of uncleanness. Zosime, who

3   Mary Douglas, 'Preface to the Routledge Classics edition', in *Purity and Danger: an Analysis of Concept of Pollution and Taboo* (1966), Routledge Classics, London, 2008, pp. xi – xiii, xiv.
4   Douglas (2008), pp. 47, 49–50. The term 'matter out of place' is frequently attributed to Mary Douglas. She cites it on p. 203 from William James, *The Varieties of Religious Experience*, London, 1952, p. 129.

was born to Greek parents in Alexandria in 1923, told me, 'we don't go to church because it is not clean for the lady. It is dirty. I couldn't explain ... don't go to church. Don't get the communion'.[5] Initially I wondered if this was due to Islamic influence in the Egyptian Greek Orthodox Church until other Greek-born women in the group concurred. Prohibition spilt over into social life for young Greek women, particularly those from peasant backgrounds, because menarche introduced a time of danger. Young women were perceived to have become a corrupting force, a threat to men in a society that stressed motherhood rather than sexuality. As a result they entered a form of bodily seclusion, wearing shapeless, concealing, clothes and a head covering, their menstrual impurity prohibiting religious activities.[6] Nor was Zosime alone in her experience. Arabic-speaking Nadia, born to Syrian and Lebanese parents in Alexandria in 1939, recalled that during menstruation 'we should not take ... accept ... from the priest [communion]'.[7] This was echoed by Maryam from Lebanon who told me, 'I am a Christian and they say that when you have your period you cannot go to church until you wash and finish properly'.[8] Later I met a group of Russian-speaking women who had recently arrived in Australia. Seda, struggling to express herself in English, told me 'I want to say about Armenian religion. Armenian religion is Gregorian, and when this period, woman with menstruation, can go into the church. Armenia and Ethiopia are Gregorian, but all Christian'.[9] However, Olena, from Ukraine, offered another view: 'Russian cannot go. Georgia, Belarus ... Orthodox'.[10] Olena provided the key – Orthodoxy. According to religious historian William E. Phipps, the third-century Bishop of Alexandria, Dionysius the Great, was the first documented leader of a Christian church to prohibit menstruating women from the Communion table on the grounds of impurity, an edict that remains upheld by church law in Eastern Orthodoxy.[11]

How did these ideas about menarche and menstruation evolve? When we consider life for women from ancient times we understand that most of their menstruating years were given to pregnancy and lactation rather

---

5   Zosime, 11, Egypt 1934.
6   Yewoubdar Beyene, *From Menarche to Menopause: Reproductive Lives of Peasant Women in Two Cultures*, State University of New York Press, Albany, 1989, p. 3.
7   Nadia, 11, Egypt 1950.
8   Maryam, 15, Lebanon 1942.
9   Seda, 14, Armenia, year unknown.
10   Olena, 11, Ukraine 1949.
11   William E. Phipps, 'The menstrual taboo in the Judeo-Christian tradition', *Journal of Religion and Health*, vol. 19, no. 4, 1980, p. 300.

than to bleeding. Consequently, the rarer the occurrence, the more profound it would have seemed, as Judith Antonelli notes.[12] In early societies the occasional menstruation would be signified by patches of blood on women's garments, on the ground where they had walked and where they reclined. We read of Rachel in Genesis, sitting in her tent on a camel's storage saddle, excusing herself to her father, 'I cannot rise up before thee; for the custom of women is upon me'.[13] Rachel may have been hiding stolen goods in the saddle and claiming 'women's custom' as an excuse, but she illustrates the reality that menstruation limited movement and made women's everyday tasks difficult. Where water was scarce, early women's skin may have borne blood in stripes down the inner thighs, under the nails, and smeared on hands and clothes. Moreover, this was blood that could not be controlled. It was messy, and humans, as Douglas persuasively argues, seek order through the control of unclean matter by taboo, which entails separation, demarcation and purification.[14]

Menarche was, and is, an anomaly, according to Douglas' theory. A young girl, neither sick nor wounded, begins to bleed. Moreover, she is neither child nor reproductive woman and this makes her place in society one of ambiguity. To the ancients this was an unstable situation, and therefore dangerous, not only to the social group around the girl but to herself, and so certain rules evolved to regulate life for the menarcheal girl during her first period and in diverse ways, according to her culture, with subsequent menstruation.[15] When working as a midwife I occasionally encountered the menstruating newborn girl. This is a fine example of anomaly but one missing in the anthropological literature I have read, so the meaning associated with it in traditional societies remains unknown.[16] When the ambiguous and the anomalous become part of the religious belief system, clear rules are drawn between the sacred and the secular and transgressions are punished.

---

12   Judith Antonelli, *In the Image of God: a Feminist Commentary on the Torah*, Jason Aronson Inc. New Jersey, 1997, p. 287. Deborah Winslow also suggests that infrequency of menstruation may increase tensions surrounding menarche. See Deborah Winslow, 'Rituals of first menstruation in Sri Lanka', *Man*, vol. 15, no. 4, 1980, p. 623 f.n. 21.
13   'Genesis', 31:35, *The Holy Bible*, King James' version, Cambridge University Press, Cambridge n.d.
14   Douglas (2008), p. 5.
15   Buckley and Gottlieb in Buckley and Gottlieb (eds), (1988), p. 7.
16   The phenomenon of infant menstruation is caused by the withdrawal, at birth, of the maternal oestrogen that the foetus has been exposed to in the womb. See Margaret Myles, *Textbook for Midwives*, Churchill Livingstone, Edinburgh 1975, p. 450.

The concept of danger is heard in Cecile's story. Cecile comes from a village in Uganda and was away from home at the time of her menarche. She spoke hesitantly of another concern: 'I was staying in another place with an auntie … but I didn't tell her because I was told she might do something … or even … especially that first thing is very important'.[17] Cecile was alluding to the power associated with menarcheal blood. She had been warned not to let that power get into the wrong hands. She went on carefully: 'also, because we didn't have pads … we were using cloth … from old linens … the first thing you used you give to your mum and that's…' Cecile laughed with embarrassment '…but I don't know what they did with it'. Cecile had shared as much as she wanted to on that subject. I found the same with Ruth, also from Uganda, a deeply religious woman who was at boarding school at the time of her menarche. When asked about any traditional responses to menarche in her culture, she told me, 'my mum was a Christian and, with the knowledge of Christianity which had come, she did not leave us to just go and survey things ourselves. She made a boundary for us so we had to go by those boundaries so we never … she was very cautious of these cultural events which … many of them involved the evil areas. I mean all the superstitions which are totally not in line with Christianity … we were protected from that so we never had experience of them at all. Most of the cultural things are truly very wicked and cause a lot of fear'.[18] These two women, both from cultures where traditional belief systems are seemingly at odds with modernity and Christianity, experienced menarche during the escalating civil wars that followed Ugandan independence (in 1962) – a time when many thousands of women were becoming victims of rape.[19] Cecile introduces the concept of menarcheal blood and power and Ruth's denial of knowledge confirms its existence, together with the inference of danger. I was reminded of anthropologist Alma Gottlieb's findings among the West African Beng, many of whom are now Islamic or Christian, but still take part in some of the older traditional belief practices, such as using menstrual blood for witchcraft with the intention of affecting others in either positive or negative ways.[20]

---

17 Cecile, 16, Uganda 1965.
18 Ruth, 17, Uganda c.1974.
19 Helen Liebling-Kalifani, Angela Marshall, Ruth Ojiambo-Ochieng, and Nassozi Margaret Kakembo, 'Experiences of women war-torture survivors in Uganda: implications for health and human rights', *Journal of International Women's Studies*, vol. 8, no. 4, 2007, pp. 1–2.
20 Alma Gottlieb, 'Menstrual cosmology among the Beng of Ivory Coast', in Buckley and Gottlieb (eds), (1988), p. 56. See Buckley and Gottlieb in Buckley and Gottlieb (eds), (1988), p. 35.

So it was that Cecile protected her now-ambiguous self from the anomaly of menarche, that of the power of first blood, by concealing it from a woman who might cause harm. Ruth was protected from the inferred danger of traditional practices by her mother's Christian boundaries. For the Greek and Russian-speaking women following the Eastern and Russian Orthodox belief systems, there was compliance with ancient rules of Leviticus, inevitably quoted in studies of menstrual exclusion.

Before Christianity and Islam, Leviticus had long provided Jewish women with laws directing menstrual conduct. These commandments have been regarded by feminists as a template for women's oppression by men, and by others as a hygiene guide for avoiding contagion.[21] Because Leviticus is enormously influential in the lives of so many women, I include the relevant verses here:

> She shall be put apart seven days: and whoever toucheth her shall be unclean until the evening.

> Everything that she lieth upon in her separation shall be unclean: everything also that she sitteth upon shall be unclean.

> Whoever toucheth her bed shall wash his clothes, and bathe himself in water, and be unclean until the even.

> And if it be on her bed, or on anything whereon she sitteth, when he toucheth it, he shall be unclean until the even.

> And if any man lie with her at all, and her flowers be upon him, he shall be unclean seven days; and all the bed whereon he lieth shall be unclean.

> But if she be cleansed of her issue, then she shall number to herself seven days, and after that she shall be clean.

> And on the eighth day she will take unto her two turtles, or two young pigeons, and bring them to the priest, to the door of the tabernacle.

---

21 See Janice Delaney, Mary Jane Lupton and Emily Toth, 'Women unclean: menstrual taboos in Judaism and Christianity', in *The Curse: a Cultural History of Menstruation* (1976), University of Illinois Press, Urbana, 1988, pp. 37–38, 48–49. See also Tova Hartman and Naomi Marmon, 'Lived regulations, systemic attributions: menstrual separation and ritual immersion in the experience of Orthodox Jewish women', *Gender and Society*, vol. 18, no. 3, 2004, pp. 389–390. Liubov (Louba) Ben-Noun indicates the roots of preventative medicine may be seen in Leviticus in 'What is the biblical attitude towards personal hygiene during vaginal bleeding?', *European Journal of Obstetrics and Gynaecology and Reproductive Biology*, vol. 106, no. 1, 2003, pp. 99–101.

And the priest shall offer the one for a sin offering, and the other for a burnt offering; and the priest shall make an atonement for her before the Lord for the issue of her uncleanness.[22]

The ambiguity of women's blood has an added dimension in Leviticus: that of the power and danger of contagion. By assigning the problem to the sacred, the mechanism of defence and protection is enacted under the aegis of divine authority. Women are separated and demarcated in the secular space and prohibited from the sacred until purification and atonement are obtained through animal blood sacrifice.

Leviticus remained the authoritative text in the Western Christian tradition until the sixth century, and women continued to be prohibited from entering the church or taking communion. In 596 CE Augustine, first bishop of the Catholic Church in England, wrote to the Pope to ask about women's menstrual exclusion from church. The Pope's response reflected a change of thought based on the Gospels:

A woman should not be forbidden to enter church during these times, for the workings of nature cannot be considered culpable, and it is not just that she should be refused admittance, since her condition is beyond her control. We know that the woman who suffered an issue of blood, humbly approaching behind our Lord, touched the hem of his robe, and was at once healed of her sickness ... A woman, therefore, should not be forbidden to receive the mystery of Communion at these times. If any out of a deep sense of reverence do not presume to do so, this is commendable; but if they do so, they do nothing wrong. For while the Old Testament makes outward observances important, the New Testament does not regard these things so highly as the inward disposition, which is the sole true criterion. Therefore ... how can a woman who endures the laws of nature with a pure mind be considered impure?[23]

However, medieval historian Monica Green points out that Pope Gregory's attempts to bring about change did not have unanimous support within the

---

22 'Leviticus', 15:19–24, 15: 28–30, *Holy Bible*, King James version, Cambridge University Press, Cambridge, n.d.

23 'The letter of Pope Gregory' 1.27, in *Bede: A History of the English Church and People* trans. Leo Sherley-Price, Penguin Books, Middlesex, 1956, pp. 78–79. For the description of Christ reacting to the touch of the bleeding woman see Luke 8: 43–48, *Holy Bible* King James version. See also Charles T. Wood. 'The doctor's dilemma: sin, salvation, and the menstrual cycle in medieval thought', *Speculum*, vol. 56, no. 4, 1981, p. 713–714. Wood notes that the term 'nature' is used in reference to the infirm state of humanity after the Fall.

church. As a result the prohibition remained until the 12th century, when Pope Innocent III affirmed the earlier decree of Pope Gregory, allowing a menstruating woman to stay out of church but not prohibiting her attendance – a shift in religious thought that effected cultural change.[24]

This divergence from the Eastern Orthodox tradition altered the concept of menarcheal and menstrual uncleanness by transferring the source of impurity from the body to the mind. Thus, in Western Christian churches, the Levitical prohibition of the menarcheal and menstruating woman entering the sacred space and receiving communion became, and remained, invalid. Over eight centuries later, the responses of elderly Italian-born women to the question about menarche, and attitudes of the Roman Catholic Church toward it, were hardly unexpected. Loretta had quickly replied that at menarche and thereafter she could attend church when menstruating, 'yes, yes, that's a ... that's nature. There's no harm. That's nature'.[25] Neve brought a certain authority to her response, arguing 'I have two uncles who are priests. Nobody say this'.[26] However, Ramona, a Spanish-speaking Chilean woman, introduced another aspect to my question about religion and menarche – virginity as a metaphor for purity. For Ramona the remembered connection between menarche and her Roman Catholicism was her struggle with the mind–body imperatives that her developing sexuality caused, 'because you have to go in a white and virgin to the church anytime you get married'.[27] Her emphasis on the significance of virginity was reiterated by the other Chilean women, suggesting a further shift in thought from menstrual uncleanness to the religious model of purity provided by the Virgin Mary, akin to the idealised feminine identity constructed by male priests in late medieval England, as we saw in chapter one.

Yet for women of Orthodox Jewish belief, Leviticus remains the main authority. Yanuva, who was born in Egypt in 1946 to Sephardic parents, experienced menarche while in transit as a refugee from Nasser's regime. She explained that her mother's Sephardic heritage embraced a Kabbalistic

24 Monica H. Green, 'Flowers, poisons and men: menstruation in medieval Western Europe', in *Menstruation: a Cultural History*, Andrew Shail and Gillian Howie (eds), Palgrave Macmillan, Basingstoke, 2005, pp. 59–60. Winslow (1980) refers to Vatican II reiterating Pope Gregory's dictum that menstruating women should not be barred from attending church. Winslow (1980) notes that among Sri Lankan Catholics the perception of uncleanness remained into the 1970s and women chose to absent themselves, p. 623 f.n. 19. This tradition may have reflected Buddhist and Hindu influences.
25 Loretta, 10, Italy 1947.
26 Neve, 11, Italy 1941.
27 Ramona, 15, Chile 1964.

tradition, and that 'the main focus of a synagogue is the ark and it's like a cupboard, and inside the cupboard are the Torah scrolls, and three times a week … Mondays, Thursdays, Saturdays, a Torah scroll is taken out and we read from it. OK? So, when the Torah scroll is out you're not, according to my mother, you're not allowed to look at it. So you have to keep your face down, or up, or turn your face away because you are not allowed to look at it because it's too holy … and that can translate itself to not even to go to synagogue when you've got your periods … and the other thing is, in the regular run-of-the-mill Jewish law … when the wife within the family is menstruating, and for a week afterwards, she is called Niddah, and they separate. You don't have any physical contact, definitely no sexual contact. You can't even lift the same object which means you can't hand a child from one to the other. You can't hand anything over from one to the other'.[28] The significance of Niddah for Jewish women is present in Yanuva's brief reference and I was interested to discover, some time later, that today's Jewish girls attend special weekly classes over the course of a year, from when they are about 11, in preparation for their Bat Mitzvah, the religious coming-of-age at the age of 12. In place of learning Torah, as their male counterparts do, some synagogues place the emphasis on learning how to become good Jewish women and mothers. The girls are instructed in the women's role for Shabbat and other rituals, and learn about Niddah, or ritual purity, including visiting a micveh, the traditional Jewish women's immersion bath through which purification is achieved after menstruation. For girls from less religious backgrounds, attending non-Jewish schools, this may be the only religious education specific to Jewish women and women's bodies they will receive.[29]

At the time of menarche Yanuva was more concerned with learning how to manage her menstrual cloths, made by her mother, which she had to wash according to her mother's interpretation of Jewish law. 'You would soak it in the sun for 24 hours and you would get down on your hands and knees and scrub it, and you weren't allowed to pour the water … like you weren't allowed to do it in the sink because as far as my mother was concerned it was spiritually impure and had to go in the toilet. So you had to do it outside … on the ground. It was like a whole story'. In this recollection, Yanuva puts the practical face to Jewish law. When asked about food preparation when menstruating Yanuva replied, 'that's interesting because I think …

---

28   Yanuva, 10, Egypt, 1957.
29   'Mazel Tov! Mazel Tov! Bar and Bat Mitzvah', *Compass*, ABC 1, Sunday 16 August 2009.

I think there's something there that I don't even remember. Nowadays I don't think it applies because a woman in Niddah still has to cook for her family, but in the olden days when they lived around a courtyard with an extended family there was always a grandmother or an older sister or cousin or somebody who wouldn't mind to cook and therefore they were able not to touch the food. Definitely if you're talking about the Temple Era then there were certain things that a woman could not touch'.[30]

Niddah today is a ritualised practice governing sexual relations in marriage. The practice had greater significance to the menarcheal girl before the destruction of the First and Second Temples in 560 BCE and 70 CE, because her impurity, or *tumat niddah*, prohibited her from crossing the boundary into the Temple and from touching food and utensils used in religious worship.[31] This is what Yanuva was referring to. During the time of the Second Temple, a girl who would become known as the Virgin Mary reached her religious coming-of-age at 12, creating a problem for the priests who asked what they could do to prevent her polluting the Temple. The answer was betrothal to Joseph.[32] But it was not Mary per se that was the problem. Rather it was the ambiguity of the child's body in a situation which Charlotte Elisheva Fonrobert describes as the forensic context. Referring to the Babylonian Talmud, Fonrobert observes that potential menarche created the dividing line between purity and impurity, with associated unease about Temple pollution. Before menarche a girl was in a state of purity and might handle Temple items without cause for concern. Between 11 years and one day and 12 years and one day, she was considered under *halakhah* (religious law) to be approaching her season, her legal coming-of-age, and was in a state of presumptive impurity, with pending menarche causing anxiety over her handling of Temple items. As her bodily blood was believed to be increasing in readiness to breach the boundary, a prior examination was carried out for the purpose of advance recognition of bleeding and its concomitant change of status. In this, Fonrobert suggests rabbinical participation, whether or not with awareness of Roman and other ancient cultures, in a legal discourse on the young female body, although for Jewish practice the examination was primarily to protect Temple-related items from impurity.[33] After destruction

---

30 Yanuva, 10, Egypt 1957.
31 Haviva Ner-David, 'Medieval *responsa* literature on Niddah: perpetuations of notions of *tumah*', in Shail and Howie (eds), (2005), p. 188.
32 Wood (1981), p. 722.
33 Charlotte Elisheva Fonrobert, *Menstrual Purity: Rabbinic and Christian Reconstructions of Biblical Gender*, Stanford University Press, Stanford California, 2000, pp. 137–143. See also f.n. 19, p. 269.

of the Second Temple the need for these strictures was removed and Niddah became solely concerned with religious law regarding sexual relations.[34]

Religious law and its interpretation relating to menarche and menstruation, as my interviewees described, continued the theme of uncleanness. I met with two groups of women from the youngest of the monotheistic religions, Islam, who added their voices. The women were culturally very different as one group were Arabic-speakers from Lebanon and the other from Indonesia. The Indonesian group from Java, wearing Western dress, explained their belief was mixed, syncretic, as Islam overlaid the older *abangan* animist tradition. By contrast the Lebanese women wore Islamic dress and Rashida explained through an interpreter that 'when she has a period she is not allowed to go to the mosque to pray. She must stay home and she is not allowed to touch the Qur'an, the holy book, until the seven days she will wash herself well. There is nothing that cannot be washed'.[35] This was echoed by Nirmala, from Jogjakarta, who reminded me that not entering the mosque 'is always sort of general for Muslim people, you know that, as I said you don't go to do praying ... we don't fast because they consider you have period you are in a dirty'. Wani interrupted, 'but also because you are losing blood'. Nirmala continued, 'when we finish period we always have to drink jamu, a herbal medicine to cleanse, and also when we finish we have to wash our hair, then you would be allowed to do praying and also during the fasting month you're allowed to fast'.[36] Moroccan sociologist Fatima Mernissi notes that religious education for a Muslim starts with attention to the body: the orifices, secretions and fluids that the child must learn to monitor and control. Girls learn that they must wash their bodies according to a strict ritual after menstruating.[37] Once again, we see the boundaries of the sacred enacted through religiously prescribed seclusion, demarcation and purification, acting as a defence and protection (for others) from the impurity of menarche and subsequent menstruation.

Islam attributes the uncleanness of women to Eve, an ambiguous figure that determines constructions and perceptions of gender in Judaism and

---

34 See Jonah Steinberg, 'From a "pot of filth" to a "hedge of roses" (and back): changing theorizations of menstruation in Judaism', *Journal of Feminist Studies in Religion*, vol. 13, no. 2, 1997, pp. 8–9. The Second Temple was destroyed by Roman legions.

35 Rashida, 14, Lebanon, year unknown.

36 Nirmala, 13, Indonesia 1964.

37 Fatima Mernissi, *Women and Islam: an Historical and Theological Enquiry*, trans. Mary Jo Lakeland, Women Unlimited Press, New Delhi, 2004, p. 74.

Christianity.[38] According to historian D. A. Spellberg, the interpretation of Eve was revised as Muslim scholars selected certain existing written and oral sources from the older monotheistic traditions in the establishment of Islam, the writing of the Qur'an, and the life of the prophet Muhammad. Thus Adam became the first of a chain of 24 prophets ending with Muhammad who, through Allah, perfected the content of the Torah and Gospels. We learn that Adam and his unnamed female companion were created by Allah from one soul. Spellberg tells us Allah warned Adam and his companion, addressing them as a single entity, about the forbidden tree in the garden, and the enmity of Satan. They are tempted by Satan as a couple, after which Satan tempts Adam alone, but they eat the prohibited fruit together. Their mutual repentance follows their recognition of shared responsibility for their shame but fails to prevent their punishment by expulsion from paradise.[39]

This Qur'anic version of the Fall was reinterpreted by Muslim scholars during the establishment of an Islamic tradition. Religious historians Jane Smith and Yvonne Haddad argue that Islamic commentators ignored the construction of Eve in the Qur'anic version, repeatedly returned to the biblical narrative that represented Eve as the cause for Adam's fall.[40] Spellberg points out that although women had no part in writing the Qur'an, they are acknowledged as contributors to Islamic *isnāds*, the authoritative oral testimony preceding every distinct rendering of *hadith* (the reported sayings and doings of Muhammad). Writers of the final collection of data included Al-Tabari (d.923), whose hadith-like format was prefaced by isnād allowing construction of Eve, including a version attributed to Ibn Ishaq (d.767). Ibn Ishaq, an early biographer of the prophet Muhammad, merged collected material from Judaic and Christian sources as the Muslim Companions of the Prophet had been instructed to do. As a result, Al-Tabari's Eve reflects Genesis in her creation from Adam's rib rather than his soul, and she is named Hawwa, meaning Eve. Her agent in duplicity is a female snake who allows Satan, or Iblis, the fallen angel, entry to her body for passage into the

---

38 'Genesis', 2:21–24, 3:22, *Holy Bible*, King James' version, Cambridge University Press, Cambridge n.d.

39 D. A. Spellberg, 'Writing the unwritten life of the Islamic Eve: menstruation and the demonization of motherhood', *International Journal of Middle East Studies*, vol. 28, no. 3, 1996, pp. 306–307. In their paper 'Eve: Islamic image of woman', Jane I. Smith and Yvonne Haddad indicate three other places in the Qur'an where the single soul is stated to be the source of creation of both man and his mate, but these are the only references to the creation of woman. See *Women's Studies International Forum*, vol. 5, no. 2, 1982, p. 136.

40 Smith and Haddad (1982), p. 138.

banned garden. Having slunk into paradise (at that time the snake still had legs), Satan/Iblis successfully urges Eve to eat the forbidden fruit after which Eve persuades Adam. According to Spellberg, this is the Islamic rendering of the Fall, even though the Qur'an describes Satan/Iblis enticing Adam alone.[41]

With the ambiguity of Eve's responses to Satan, further explanation of her character was developed through a section of hadith written by Ibn Maja (d.888), which relates to ritual purity in the care of urinating children. Here it is written that the Prophet said the boy should be wet and the girl cleansed. This instruction was further interpreted by legal scholar al-Shafi'I (d.820) as meaning that boys were made from the same material as their progenitor, Adam, who had been created from clay and water. However, as Eve was created from Adam's short rib, girls were made from Eve's flesh and blood. But Genesis tells us Eve was made from Adam's 'flesh and bone' and in the Qu'ran, Adam is made from clay, or mud, and Eve is created from his soul. The introduction of blood as Eve's forming substance immediately introduces the concept of impurity and of women being born unclean and essentially different from men. At menarche this impurity becomes ritualised in Islamic practice, a constant reminder of Eve, who caused the tree in the garden to bleed, and was punished by Allah, through the generations, with menstruation.[42]

From the People of the Book I moved to Buddhist traditions, meeting Nila, Keshini and Daksha from Sri Lanka. Keshini recognised her menarche on waking, remembering 'my mother saw it in the morning and she kept me inside, then she called the washing woman we call dhobi and she came and she showered me and she gave me her clothes then, from there onwards, I used to wear the clothes that she brings because we had to give everything, including my gold earrings, to dhobi. We are not supposed to keep any of the things that we had on our body. Even this gold ... I had very beautiful gold earrings with some pink colour stone, I can't remember the name of the stone, it was a very good one, and I loved them and I can remember I didn't want to give, but we're not supposed to keep them, you know? We gave everything. Even my mother was a bit, you know, she was worried because of course, precious ... something precious ... some people change their earrings when they are at that stage ... you know? I had very good ones but my mother couldn't help it and she had to give them away. After that

41   Spellberg (1996), pp. 308–309, 311–312.
42   Spellberg (1996), p. 313.

immediately the dhobi came and gave me a bath. I can't remember if it was a special auspicious time or not but after that I wasn't allowed to see any of my brothers, or my father, or any man. I was in the room all the time and food and everything were brought to the room, and even I go to the toilet and they are sitting there, they just go away, you know? My mother says now I am coming and no one stays'.[43]

Daksha had noticed blood on her clothes as she prepared for bed and told her mother, receiving a similar response to Keshini: 'she said you can wait today but you must go to your room, and when it was daytime my mother brings the dhobi woman and we had to remove everything. Seven days inside the house, can't see anybody, can't go out, everything is inside. We have the bathing, get the horoscope, take the date to do the ceremony'.[44] Daksha's story was interrupted before she could finish, but confirmed a commonality in the Sri Lankan Buddhist experience of menarche, although I wondered what menarche meant for young girls in a tradition in which rebirth as a woman was a backward step or bad karma. In the search for answers I found that Prince Siddhārtha, the future Buddha, had been repulsed by the bodies of women whose impurity was evident in menstruation.[45] But, by the time of transformation, his teachings emphasised a philosophy that was both gender neutral and gender exclusive, according to feminist Buddhist scholar Rita Gross. While Buddhist scholar Alan Sponberg agrees, he points out the teachings were not without orthodox criticism, particularly toward radical ideas about women's capacity for spirituality which remained within a framework of cultural assumptions.[46] Gross observes that the place of women in Buddhism is frequently told in the stories of the Earth Goddess who responded to Siddhārtha Gautama's plea for a witness to his many good deeds in earlier lifetimes. Her willingness helped him attain enlightenment as the Buddha and illustrates how women are necessary in every context of Buddhism. However, the context for women remained one of domestic labour interspersed with devotional practices including provision of food for the monks in an environment of close contact between the monastic

---

43   Keshini, 12, Sri Lanka 1969.
44   Daksha, 13, Sri Lanka 1947.
45   Julia Leslie, 'Some traditional Indian views on menstruation and female sexuality', in *Sexual Knowledge, Sexual Science: the History of Attitudes to Sexuality,* Roy Porter and Mikuláš Teich (eds), Cambridge University Press, Cambridge, 1994, pp. 69–70.
46   Rita M. Gross, 'Buddhism', in *Her Voice, Her Faith: Women Speak Out on World Religions,* Arvind Sharma, Katherine K. Young (eds), Westview Press, Cambridge, Maryland 2002, p. 69; Alan Sponberg, 'Attitudes toward women and the feminine in early Buddhism', in *Buddhism, Sexuality, and Gender,* José Ignacio Cabezón (ed.), State University of New York Press, Albany, 1992, pp. 10–11.

and lay community (whom, initially, the Buddha taught). By the third century BCE, early Buddhist principles had spread throughout India and into Sri Lanka, incorporating much of the Indian understanding of the world, including the view of women as inferior beings, partly due to birth, and partly to the belief that women were less interested in spiritual matters. Women were perceived as unfortunate because of five woes, which included the pain of menstruation and their lack of independence due to lifelong subservience to men – fathers, husbands and sons.[47] With the concept of male dominance in women's lives, it comes as no surprise to read that Buddhist historian Bernard Faure considers Buddhism to be unremittingly misogynist, exemplified in the way existing cultural phobias about the pollutant power of women's menstrual blood became underpinned by Buddhist meaning in male thought.[48]

Specific to Sri Lankan Buddhists is the belief in *killa* – the destructive power of the menarcheal girl, against which all male members of the family must be protected, and which necessitates her seclusion. However, Swarna Wickremeratne, recalling her menarche and seclusion, related that some people believed menarche to be a time of danger to the girl herself. She was not left alone for fear she might be invaded by evil spirits in her vulnerable condition. If her companion needed to leave the room, an axe was propped against the wall as symbolic defence, inviting Swarna to reflect on her situation and on the malevolence of spirits she might be forced to defend herself against.[49] Yet there are other forms of defence. In her paper on the rituals of menarche in Sri Lanka, anthropologist Deborah Winslow points out that at this time Buddhist girls may relate especially to the female goddess Pattinī, whose birth from a mango tree created her as pure, and whose powers of protection and destruction make her a goddess of contrasts. At menarche, when the young girl's *killa* becomes more dangerous to others than at the time of giving birth or at death, she may be thought to represent the fearful, virginal powers of Pattinī.[50] It is in this duality that the community perceives a threat to cosmic purity, according to anthropologists Thomas Buckley and Alma Gottlieb.[51]

47   Gross in Sharma and Young (eds) (2003), pp. 59–61, 63–65, 88–89.
48   Bernard Faure, *The Power of Denial: Buddhism, Purity, and Gender,* Princeton University Press, New Jersey, 2003, pp. 9, 66.
49   Swana Wickremeratne, *Buddhism in Sri Lanka: Remembered Yesterdays,* State University of New York Press, Albany, 2006, pp. 78–79.
50   Winslow (1980), pp. 615–617.
51   Buckley and Gottlieb in Buckley and Gottlieb (eds), (1988), p. 10.

Threats of the destructive powers of menarche were absent in interviews with two other Buddhist women, both Chinese-Vietnamese. They had both experienced menarche at a time of national conflict and profound social instability and how much this influenced perceptions of socio-religious life is unknown. In contrast to the Sri Lankan interviewees, neither knew of any menarcheal ritual in the Buddhist tradition, but both were aware of menstrual impurity. When asked about temple attendance Bao had responded 'aieee, no. No go in. We are [unclean] when we've got the period. Don't go, that's rude'.[52] Her friend, Tu, added 'before we not go, but some old lady said "don't worry", because she asked why we didn't go, and we said we're dirty, and she said "don't worry you can go anytime because this one the Buddha give you. It's natural. All the girls have this"'.[53] I was interested in the difference between the Sri Lankan tradition of seclusion and ritual and its absence among Chinese-Vietnamese, and also in the suggestion made by the older woman – possibly no longer menstruating therefore free of pollution – that bodily function was not unclean, a statement with clear overtones of Pope Gregory. The belief that menstruation was a gift from the Buddha suggests some other cultural influence, possibly the French Catholicism of colonialism. I discovered that among the bodhisattvas (those striving for perfect enlightenment in order to benefit all sentient beings),[54] an Indian male, Avalokiteśvara, had been transformed into a beautiful Chinese woman known as Kuan-Yin, who is always represented in white. Kuan-Yin symbolises women's problems, including those associated with menstruation, and is attributed to helping Chinese women free themselves from culturally defined gender restrictions.[55] Anthropologist Steven Sangren, examining the connection between women's social roles and pollution beliefs in Chinese religious symbols, suggests a certain juxtaposition with female deities. Consequently, if Kuan-Yin is to symbolise the feminine ideal she must be free from the pollution of menarcheal and menstrual blood. Because of her pure state, Kuan-Yin protects women from ritual impurity, therefore women entering Kuan-Yin temples to recite their daily Buddhist sutras see the activity as one of purification.[56] Under such conditions Bao and Tu, as

---

52   Bao, 12, Vietnam 1968.
53   Tu, 14, Vietnam 1963.
54   Gross in Sharma and Young (eds) (2003), pp. 70–71.
55   Barbara Reed, 'The gender symbolism of Kuan-yin bodhisattva', in *Buddhism, Sexuality, and Gender*, José Ignacio Cabezón (ed.), State University of new York Press, Albany, 1992, p. 159.
56   P. Steven Sangren, 'Female gender in Chinese religious symbols: Kuan Yin, Ma Tsu, and the "eternal mother"', *Signs*, vol. 9, no. 1, 1983, pp. 4, 11–12.

menstruants, may have been able to enter temples dedicated to a female bodhisattva without fear of spiritual uncleanness.

Menarcheal and menstrual impurity is part of the Hindu religious belief system. My interviewees included Hindu women from Sri Lanka, India and Kenya, each with a story containing shades of difference that the Indian women explained was due to variation in religious practice from state to state. Nila had recalled being 'very nervous, and immediately I told my mother I was isolated because I was not supposed to see my father. They kept me private, and then they did tell all my family members, like my close aunties and uncles and the ladies and then I think, on that day itself, the ladies ... I think it was my grandma and my aunties, three or four, I can't remember, they gave me a bath ... on the day itself. It was blessed and they each took turn to pour the water and after that I just showered myself and then they gave me new clothes and I was in that room, you know? Then they go and look at the time, that particular time, and the date was very significant, and then they contact an astrologer or the priest, whomever, and they start to see your horoscope and apparently now, in the Hindu religion, I think it's more related to than your birth time, this time is significant in your life, in your future life, and so they look at that and I think the priest tells them, like I think it was fifteen or thirty [days] ... I'm not sure now, I can't really remember, but they say you don't go to school. I've really forgotten actually how many days it was I don't go to school, and according to the priest's time and everything, there's a big celebration in the family. During our periods, you know, when you have your menses, you never go and pray to God and you don't go to the temple. I personally don't agree to this because I think it's a natural thing of your body but the culture meant ... and I don't myself go to the temple. You feel, anyway, not clean in yourself. I think that makes you not want to go'.[57] Here Nila expresses the internalised belief of uncleanness and temple pollution but there is little difference in her interpretation of the menarcheal experience from that of Keshini and Daksha, an observation that bears out Deborah Winslow's study of Sri Lankan menarcheal rituals among Buddhist, Catholic, and Muslim girls, which suggested some syncretism of religious practice.[58]

Variations in Indian Hindu religious practice according to social, urban, rural and linguistic groupings complicates the interpretation of meaning for those outside their particular stratum, according to Hindu scholar Kartikeya

---

57   Nila, 13, Sri Lanka 1964.
58   Winslow (1980), p. 604.

Patel, who observes that Hinduism is not one tradition but an overarching term incorporating many traditions.[59] The women interviewed represented variation, both in experience and attitude. Netri told me 'we were quite a broad-minded family. No, you don't go to temples during that, but even that my mother never said, you know. It's not a big deal ... and they didn't do worship and those things. My mother, I think, didn't do that',[60] but Hettal remembered a different experience. 'When I had my period no go to temple and no worshipping in home also. I can't enter this room, because in India everywhere one room is special for God, but I can't touch it and not touch food also because my grandma told me is separate. No, don't touch. Sometimes I see only four days I can't go to room but fifth day also bleeding but can go. It's questionable. Sometimes fifth day, sixth day bleeding is over but not allowed. If I touch the water, my aunties they not take this water. After three days allow you to touch water'.[61] Hetal's understandable scepticism over the time she is considered impure is reinforced by Hindu scholar David Smith's explanation that purity/impurity is not altogether physical, arguing the menarcheal girl's second bath on the fifth day purifies her even though she may still be bleeding, and if her bleeding ceases before the fifth day she remains impure until she has the second bath.[62] Thus the symbolism of time determining purity/impurity is as ambiguous as the menarche that caused it. Moreover, although Hettal is very clear about prohibition of entry to the domestic shrine from the time of menarche, anthropologist Karin Kapadia draws attention to families who worship lineage deities that are not offended by menarcheal impurity of a girl from the household. They are, however, affronted by the menarcheal pollution of an outsider.[63] So it would appear Hettal's position in the household was that of an outsider. Certainly, her 'aunties' regarded her as contagiously impure. Again, the ambiguity of menarche is symbolised by a concept of danger which Kapadia considers to be caused by the unpredictability of planetary influences. Hettal was vulnerable at this time of transformation from child to adult, and the domestic prohibitions she experienced were structured responses to the anomaly of her menarcheal blood, its power and her vulnerability to that power.[64]

---

59   Kartikeya C. Patel, 'Women, earth, and the goddess: a Shākta-Hindu interpretation of embodied religion, *Hypatia*, vol. 9. no. 4, 1994, p. 71.

60   Netri, 14, India 1951.

61   Hetal, 14, India c.1952.

62   David Smith, *Hinduism and Modernity*, Blackwell Publishing, Oxford, 2003, p. 111.

63   Karin Kapadia, *Siva and her Sisters: Gender, Caste, and Class in Rural South India*, Westview Press, Boulder, 1995, p. 96.

64   Kapadia (1995), p. 101.

Hindu belief related to the power of menarche differed in time and place, as Karuna relates. 'I was going to a village school but that was a different sect, much more reformed than some of the ones that are connected to temples, and the principal of that school was also such that, if in a Hindu temple there were some restrictions, he said "no". He was only fourteen I think, and he was sitting for pudja, when you are praying for certain gods in front of a fire. There was a little candle burning, and there was food around it, and this was a holy thing, and he was sitting all night without sleeping, and he was fasting. That food was supposed to be pure, and a little mouse came in the middle of the night, and nibbled at that food, and the fellow changed in that moment. He said "if a little mouse can come and nibble out of that food which people consider very holy and it's right in front of the god … he said I'm not going to worry about this religion" and he reformed so many things. He said girls should get an education as well as boys. They should be equal to boys. And that was the reason he started this school, built specially for girls, in 1937 and I was five when I joined that school, one of the first ones. They said [menstruation] was natural. You see? It was natural and it has to come. In some religions you can't go to the temple and if you have your period you can't fast. You're not allowed to because you're not pure or clean … but my teacher just said "it's natural"'.[65] After hearing Karuna's story I read of another reform that occurred in India during the mid-1970s, in the temple of Adi Para Shakti (the Primordial Great Powerful Goddess), situated in the village of Mel Maruvattur some distance from Madras. A young man of the village experienced a revelation that the goddess was present and that she wanted it known that her followers were equal, regardless of gender, race or caste, because they shared the same red blood. This was to be symbolised by the wearing of red when people visited the temple to worship her. Furthermore, menstruating women were to be included.[66] In both these stories the revelations occurred to young men, each acting as an agent of change affecting young women. Each man created a liberal environment for girls' education and worship that removed traditional religious strictures toward menarche and menstruation.

Liberation from the prohibitions of Hindu tradition was very much on Alisha's mind when I interviewed her. She has seen and experienced a great deal, having been born in Madras in 1929, and she spoke of responses

---

65 Karuna, Kenya, age and year of menarche unknown.
66 Vasudha Narayanan, 'Hinduism', in *Her Voice, Her Faith: Women Speak on World Religions*, Arvind Sharma and Katherine K. Young (eds), Worldview Press, Cambridge, Maryland, 2002, pp. 46–47.

to the impurity of menarche according to Hindu belief in the framework of India's dowry system. Initially it seemed distant from the subject of menarche but the historic implications for girls became clear. She told me that 'girls were actually regarded as weeds in the garden because a girl means, in those days, dowry, and people cannot afford to have dowry and they have to sell their property, lose jobs, borrow, go into debts, and one daughter, significant difficulty. So when you have two, three daughters the man will have to go with a begging bowl after that, for they insist on dowry. They were not ... women were not educated. But this dowry business – they start setting up from the time the child is born. A girl is unwanted. If there's a boy in the house they give the cream of the milk to that boy and the watery milk to the girl. That's the treatment they had in my days. And it is very seldom that we get the affection of both father and mother because mother, she actually was in the shadow of the father. The wife, the wife has no say in anything. What the husband says, she has to listen; and they are not supposed to mix with the others ... but mostly in the remote areas if they find out they have another girl they kill that child even when it is in the foetal state; and after it is born also, they think it is ... like a religious duty that she should be destroyed if it's a girl. Many have done it. But the dowry is the curse. Because of that only they're not wanted. Girl ... they have to protect the girl. So, by the time the girl is about ten, eleven, they have to look for a husband ... sometimes even five. My grandmother was only five years old. My grandfather ten years. They were married. Soon after the marriage they started fighting for one banana. That was the state in those days. Then, as for the periods, they never told us anything. They didn't guide us. But they thought ... that was another taboo ... to talk to a girl about it later and ... about marriage and first night and all. They don't talk because, like they said at the time, they'll talk to the girls later. So that type of education is not given to the girls. So they're ignorant. So when they get their first period, supposed they are they are in school or playing with the children, they think they're finished, they will die. They didn't know what exactly it was. So they come home, with bleeding on clothes, and then they are put aside. Maybe for three days, not allowed to see anyone and just kept away segregated from the family. Kept separate because nobody can go near her [because] she's considered impure. Separate bedding, one mat will be given her and some rags would be given. She's not allowed to come out from anywhere. Back door. In the villages they've got this habit: they make a hole and make the child sit there. They don't even give napkins. No sanitary pads. They were not even known in those days. The villagers are just like that and ... then, after that, she's given bath and they'll be celebration. That celebration is like an announcement that there's a girl ready for marriage. Once the girl attains puberty she's ready for wedlock'.[67]

Both historically and religiously, menarche was a public statement of readiness either for marriage, or for consummation if the marriage has taken place in childhood, as it had for Alisha's grandmother. We know from chapter one that in ancient Greek and Roman cultures, early defloration of girls was practised for physiological reasons. Hindus believed in it because of concepts of women's sexuality and impurity. Patel argues that the concepts of the feminine and menstruation are not only inseparable, but part of religious tradition. According to Patel, the term *dharmaritu* combines two notions: *dharma* meaning religion and *ritu,* meaning both menstruation and seasonal cycles and changes, as well as cosmic order, although strictly speaking, ritu refers to the time of post-menstrual purification after the fourth day, believed to begin the season of fertility. But dharma has deeper meanings: it is a collection of rules to help both the individual and the collective attain human goals. Disregard for the rules can cause chaos and even destruction, and Patel stresses that menstruation is not simply biological but a framework in which human activities of significance reach fruition. Hindu scholar Barbara Holdrege reads the Hindu body as the locus of pollution, and the pure body as an ideal to be constantly sought in the unceasing threat to bodily boundaries, by continual entry and exit of polluted substances. Purity is reconstituted through a complex system of practices and regulations.[68] We can understand that systemic control of potential chaos becomes imperative, and we can integrate Douglas' theory of the dangers of transitional states and their anomaly and ambiguity into the Hindu menarche.

Fear about the dangers of transitional states is one of the reasons posited for child marriage. Hindu scholar Benjamin Walker explains that the entire household was put at risk if a virgin daughter reached her menarche while still under the family roof. Hindu lawgivers declared it to be sinful, the ancestors suffered torment, and the girl's parents would go to hell for their ineptitude. It was mandatory that the girl be married so that the power of

---

67   Alisha, c.14, India c.1943.
68   Patel (1994), pp. 73–73. See also Barbara A. Holdrege, 'Body connections: Hindu discourses of the body and the study of religion', *International Journal of Hindu Studies,* vol. 2, no. 3, 1998, pp. 365–366.

her menarche, her first *ritu* be properly used.[69] Proper use was the subject for long debate in 1891, following the death of a 10 or 11-year-old child from the effects of marital rape, and in the following court case and media reports Hindu orthodoxy conflicted with Indian reformers seeking to convince the colonial government to raise the age of 'consent' in marriage from 10 to 12.[70] The following newspaper excerpt, while articulating Hindu opposition, also shows the religious grounds for it:

> The performance of the garbhadhan ceremony is obligatory. Garbhadhan must be after first menstruation. It means the first cohabitation enjoined by the shastras. It is the injunction of the Hindu shastras that married girls must cohabit with their husbands on the first appearance of their menses and all Hindus must implicitly obey the injunction. And he is not a true Hindu who does not obey it ... If one girl ... menstruates before the age of twelve it must be admitted that by raising the age of consent the ruler will be interfering with the religion of the Hindus. But everyone knows that hundreds of girls menstruate before the age of twelve. And garbhas (wombs) of hundreds of girls will be tainted and impure. And thousands of children who will be born of those impure garbhas will become impure and lose their rights to offer 'pindas' [ancestral offerings].[71]

Menarche in Hinduism had become the site of religious and political struggle. It was a battle for control over power – the female power of the first ritu – by men representing different interests. It illustrates one of several facets of meaning that religious belief systems have imbued menarche with, and the social structures that organise and control the anomaly and ambiguity of menarche.

---

69   Benjamin Walker *Hindu World: an Encyclopaedic Survey of Hindus*, Indus Press, New Delhi 1995, p. 62.

70   Tanikar Sarkar, *Hindu Wife, Hindu Nation: Community, Religion, and Cultural Nationalism*, Indiana University Press, Bloomington 2001, pp. 214–215, 224–225. The age of consent was very contentious. See also Tanika Sarkar, 'A pre-history of rights: the age of consent debate in colonial Bengal', *Feminist Studies*, vol. 26, no. 3, 2000. Although the Sarda Act or Child Marriage Restraint Act of 1929 raised marriage age for girls to fourteen, religious tradition rather than Indian law still dictates child marriage for girls in parts of India. See M. Bradra, 'Changing age at marriage of girls in India', *International Journal of Anthropology*, vol. 15, nos 1–2, 2000, pp. 39, 47–48.

71   *Dainik O Samachar Chandrika*, fourteen January 1891, cited in Sarkar (2001), p. 224. Shastras are treatises forming the basis for Hindu law.

Conclusion

Interviews provided directions for further investigation into how the world's major religious belief systems constructed the menstruating body of women as unclean, and how that concept, maintained in Eastern Orthodox Christianity, Islam, Buddhism and Hinduism, continued to influence how the interviewees as young women felt about their menstruating bodies. However, there were exceptions. It was shown that where young girls had been influenced by other agents, including educated parents or educators with reforming intent, there was social transformation. Alternative knowledge acquisition shifted the authority of leadership away from the religious, with its ideas of contagion and taboo, preventing internalisation of the concept that the menstrual body as unclean.

Religious practices of exclusion and prohibition relating to menstrual uncleanness were established by interview data as part of menstrual life for many interviewees. The clear demarcation of boundaries between the purity of the sacred and the pollution of the menstruating body continued to be observed by Eastern Orthodox Christian, Islamic and some Jewish women (who avoided looking upon the sacred Torah scrolls at this time). The boundaries were clearly defined at menarche in the Sri Lankan Hindu and Buddhist traditions, with seclusion and purification ritually carried out in similar ways, but Indian Hindu observance varied according to education, region and language groupings as well as reformation within the tradition. Chinese-Vietnamese interviewees had internalised the idea of becoming unclean, and ritually practised avoidance of the sacred until given the concept of divine will in their involuntary bleeding.

Interview findings also gave some explanation for the major shifts in thinking on menstrual uncleanness in the Jewish Orthodox tradition. Further research indicated the destruction of the Second Temple caused menstrual uncleanness to become less relevant, and the concept of impurity was transferred to the ritualised practice of marital sexual relations known as Niddah. In the Western Christian tradition the historical model of menstrual uncleanness was relocated from the body to the mind, after a sixth-century papal decision declared that the involuntary nature of menstrual bleeding could not be construed as an impurity if the mind of a young woman was pure. There were no major shifts identified in Buddhism or Hinduism, although small reforms were occurring. Nonetheless, the religious context in which uncleanness is ritualised remains established in many cultures, perpetuating a particular construction of the menarcheal and menstruating body for young observers.

Chapter 4

A RATHER SPECIAL CEREMONY

I believe they want to show off a blossomed flower.[1]

From an early age, ceremony marks the special events in our social lives. Some enhance our feeling of well-being and happiness at achievement while others cause nervousness and uncertainty, perhaps even disappointment, but all take us to another level of existence where we are recognised as members of a different group. As Solon T. Kimball observed in his introduction to Arnold van Gennep's classic text *Rites of Passage*, there is no evidence that contemporary urban living has reduced the need for ritually expressing transition from one status to another.[2] Yet we have seen in chapter two that Australians from Western cultural backgrounds make no formal acknowledgement of the special event that is a girl's menarche. Indeed, most women interviewed expressed humorous surprise at the notion of ceremony associated with the first period, and they did not make any connection with certain religious or social ceremonies occurring at or about the same time. The exceptions were women from Sri Lanka, India, Indonesia and Fiji who had experienced, or witnessed, some form of ceremony.

The concept of the menarche ceremony was familiar to me, both anthropologically and through attendance at the four-day Apache menarche ceremony in New Mexico. Indeed, it was that ceremony that motivated me to seek, through my interviewees, a deeper interpretation and understanding of what the ceremony actually meant to the young subjects. Why is it still important to some cultures and what does the ceremony reveal about the broader cultural approaches to menarche? How is such a ceremony

---

1   Keshini, 12 years old at menarche, Sri Lanka 1969.
2   Solon T. Kimball, 'Introduction', in Arnold van Gennep (1908), *Rites of Passage*, trans. Monika B. Vizedom and Gabrielle L. Caffee, University of Chicago Press, Chicago 1960, p. xvii.

understood and what does it signify culturally? How is a menarche ceremony managed and by whom?

In this chapter I will argue that there are two concepts underlying the individual stories – danger and possession – and that both are also part of many cultural belief systems about menarche and are strongly associated with the need to control it. Secondly, that understanding these concepts is the key to why menarche ceremonies remain relevant among some cultural groups and not among others. As a form of comparison with menarche ceremonies in non-industrialised cultures I will argue that in Western cultures ceremonies of a religious or social nature have evolved, signifying a particular transition in the life of a young woman, which serve to indicate maturation. They are characterised by two major differences from specific menarche ceremonies: choice in participation by the young woman, and an absence of cultural belief in the dangers caused by menstruation. Where specific menarche ceremonies still exist one can see the way in which the sense of danger, posed by a menstruating woman, is linked to religious and cultural beliefs, the latter requiring male control of the menarcheal girl's potential fertility, highly valued for its power in alliance formation. (Hence the need to control access by possession of the girl's virginity until marriage has been negotiated.) By contrast, in Western societies where menarche usually occurs while girls are in school and does not in any way interrupt their schooling, it is not seen as a crucial life stage or as the prelude to immediate marriage and reproduction. These decisions, like those about virginity and fertility control, are the responsibility of the individual woman, thus removing the onset of fertility potential as grounds for a specific menarche ceremony.

Menarche ceremonies have been aptly described as rites of passage. Their purpose is one of transformation from the status of child to that of woman through a process that all participants believe affects the subject both physically and emotionally. Although ceremony may be considered through the humanities and sciences, I believe anthropological writing imparts the most comprehensive interpretations, and these will be my points of reference in this discussion.

Ceremonies can take differing forms but the early theory published in 1908 by anthropologist Arnold van Gennep continues to be influential in both approach and terminology, as anthropologist Judith Brown (1963) observed in her own work on cross-cultural rites.[3] In his best known text,

---

3   Judith Brown, 'A cross-cultural study of female initiation rites', *American Anthropologist*, new series, vol. 65, no. 4, 1963, p. 837.

Rites of Passage, van Gennep argues against anthropological and folkloric methods of extracting rites from ceremonies to be analysed in isolation, because their separation from context obscures both their meaning and purpose in the active whole.[4] Context is therefore vital to interpretation and van Gennep uses a metaphor of life as a series of passages taking the individual from one age to the next or from one social status to the next. He argues that progress through the life of each individual requires admission through certain acts and practices intended to protect society from the dangers associated with these transitions.[5] Van Gennep constructs a paradigm of tripartite acts and practices, neither uniform in significance or elaboration. These acts involve ritual separation from normal life; a liminal time of transition accompanied by special rites; and finally, the post-liminal rites that incorporate the individual in their new status.[6] It is a theory with particular relevance to menarche ceremonies because it enables clear identification of the relationship of the individual to particular socio-religious structures in a cultural context.

The publication of the English translation of van Gennep's work in 1960 brought the theory to another generation of scholars, including Mary Douglas, who found van Gennep's paradigm – in which entry to a desired room can be achieved only through dangerous passages – reflected sociological insight into the hazard of transitional states.[7] A further aspect of van Gennep's theory is the recognition of psychological change experienced by the initiate during social transformation. Anthropologists, Alice Schlegel and Herbert Barry III consider this to be the foundation stone for describing and analysing adolescent initiation ceremonies.[8] In a well-regarded study of menarche rites among Buddhists, Catholics and Muslims in Sri Lanka, anthropologist Deborah Winslow makes brief acknowledgment of van Gennep's theory and the additions others, including Douglas, have made to it in later interpretations of social structures and symbols, boundaries and margins.[9] Marla Powers applied the theory to her anthropological study on menarche ceremony as a first rite and to later

---

4   Van Gennep, trans. Vizedom and Caffee (1960), p. 89.
5   Van Gennep trans. Vizedom and Caffee (1960), pp. 2–3, 10–11.
6   Van Gennep trans. Vizedom and Caffee (1960), p. 11.
7   Mary Douglas, *Purity and Danger: an Analysis of Concept of Pollution and Taboo*, (1966), Routledge Classics, London 2008, p. 119.
8   Alice Schlegel and Herbert Barry III, 'The evolutionary significance of adolescent initiation ceremonies', *American Ethnologist*, vol. 7, no. 4, 1980, p. 696.
9   Deborah Winslow, 'Rituals of first menstruation in Sri Lanka', *Man*, vol. 15, no. 4, 1980, p. 604.

menstrual cycle rituals, arguing it facilitated both analysis and adequate explanation.[10] Van Gennep's approach has also been praised and used by the anthropologists Barbara Myerhoff, Alan Dundes, David Parkin and Thera Rasing.[11] However, not all scholars have found van Gennep's work faultless. Writing on ritual and social function, Catherine Bell is critical of van Gennep for analysing brief descriptions of rituals outside their context, although she concedes that his understanding of these activities led to further work on the relationship between ritual and social organisation and the psychological health of individuals. Bell observes that a recent consequence of van Gennep's theory is its contribution to questions asked about lack of formal rituals and the possible link with social ills in modern societies.[12] These brief sequential references to van Gennep's theory show its continued relevance to anthropological trends through the decades, having been applied to adolescent psychology through studies of menarche ceremonies in the 1970–80s, through to folkloric studies of ceremony in an attempt to give the genre a stand-alone academic profile, as a theoretical framework in studies of pre-Christian ceremonial tradition within third-world Christian communities, and in research, on the links between ceremony and mental health.

In their cross-cultural studies on menarche ceremonies, Schlegel and Barry III find greater prevalence in societies where gender identity is emphasised. In societies with increasingly complex social organisations the importance of gender is reduced, so these societies do not have menarche ceremonies. We may ask how such a ceremony is defined. Schlegel and Barry III consider ceremony as an event with social recognition of transition from childhood to the next stage, and with at least two participants, an initiate and an initiator. For them, initiation ceremonies differ from ceremonies relating to only one aspect of life, giving as an example the Jewish bar mitzvah which they argue is specific only to religious life with no broader

---

10   Mala N. Powers, 'Menstruation and reproduction: an Oglala case', *Signs*, vol. 6, no. 1, 1980, pp. 55–56.

11   Barbara Myerhoff, 'Rites of Passage' in *Celebration: Studies in Festivity and Ritual*, Victor Turner (ed.), Smithsonian Institution Press, Washington DC, 1982, p. 116; Alan Dundes, *Folklore Matters*, The University of Tennessee Press, Knoxville, 1989; David Parkin, 'Ritual as spatial direction and bodily division', in *Understanding Rituals*, Daniel de Coppet (ed.), Routledge, London, 1992, p. 23; Thera Rasing, *Passing on the Rites of Passage: Girls' Initiation Rites in the Context of an Urban Roman Catholic Community on the Zambian Copperbelt*, African Studies Centre, Leiden University, Amsterdam, 1995, pp. 34–35.

12   Catherine M. Bell, *Ritual: Perspectives and Dimensions*, Oxford, New York, 1997, pp. 35, 37.

social recognition of changed status.[13] That may be so but Rabbi Abraham Bloch defines bar mitzvah as the legal definition of an adult Jew, the secular equivalent of being *gadol* or 'grown up', a biological definition without religious significance, based on puberty rather than age.[14] It is ceremony that completes this transition although recognition as an adult would be dependent on the context of both geography and historical time.

Social activity involving others is central to menarche ceremonies – especially involving older women whose status, conferred through marriage, sexual and reproductive experience is that of the adult. Ritual and symbolism are culturally dependent, but share certain features necessary for safe transitional passage and the protection of body and mind at this time. So we see that water is used for purification, old clothing discarded and new given to symbolise the new identity, scented flowers or unguents applied to the body, gifts intended as dowry contributions, feasts and strengthening of kin alliances, and for some, marriage arrangements. The latter is the most notable difference and was absent in the lives of Sri Lankan interviewees. Conversely, the use of horoscopes to determine auspicious times for the menarche ceremony was absent in Fiji and Indonesia, indicating that cultural traditions which arise from religion can exist with later introduced beliefs in some areas but not in others. Deborah Winslow's paper on the rituals of first menstruation demonstrate that menarche ceremonies remain part of Sri Lankan Buddhist and Hindu cultures, and my interviews with Sri Lankan women confirmed many of Winslow's findings. Their descriptions establish a basis for identifying similarities and differences when compared with women's experiences in other cultures and for this reason the women's voices will be heard at some length.

According to van Gennep, seclusion is the first part of the ceremony, when the transformational change in identity begins to evolve. Keshini recalled 'they make you feel it is different now. I think that's how they let you learn. I was given the feeling if you see a man you will become uglier but if you don't see a man you will come out a pretty girl. Actually I believe they want to show off a blossomed flower because nobody sees her and after four weeks or some time you come out with different clothes. I think that's the idea anyway, to make a difference, but it changes your feelings as well. It tells you that you are grown up, and then, after that, again, the horoscope.

---

13   Alice Schlegel and Herbert Barry III, 'Adolescent initiation ceremonies: a cross-cultural code', *Ethnology*, vol. 18, no. 2, 1979, pp. 199, 206.
14   Abraham P. Bloch, *The Biblical and Historical Background of Jewish Customs and Ceremonies*, Ktav Publishing House Inc., New York, 1980, p. 19.

I'm a Buddhist. Horoscope is Hindu culture but in Sri Lanka Hinduism and Buddhism go hand-in-hand. We all have this Indian culture, you know ... and they look for a good time according to the horoscope I believe. They decide the day but I'm one hundred per cent sure that it's not as strict as Hindu culture, they do it as a sort of trend, you know?'[15]

Trend or not, the horoscope is a vital part of the menarche ceremony and one that influences its form through the setting of dates and times. To most Westerners, astrologers are star-gazers and horoscopes are an entertaining side column in the weekend papers, but in Sri Lanka the horoscope is a catalyst for every aspect of an individual's future, a mechanism by which misfortune may be foretold and avoided. Anthropologist Steven Kemper observes that the positions of astral bodies, indicated in various tables that form the textual core of astrology, acts as a system of signs and their influence over the individual is a technology that accords with Sinhalese understanding of the self and each other within their society. Kemper provides a brief historical background explaining how a specifically Sinhalese form of astrology emerged in the second half of the 13th century when Anomadassi, a Buddhist monk whose contribution to astrological literature was significant, wrote the *Daivajñakāmadhenu*.[16] Sri Lankan political, state, and Buddhist institutions are guided by astrology in setting times for notable activities. Less public is the notable activity surrounding the menarcheal girl. Kemper suggests astrology can be constructed as a cultural category of 'individual' and 'time'. Hence, to an astrologer the individual is simply matter containing the code for its own development, and time is the variable stimulus. Therefore individuals exist only so far as they exist in time. Change can be brought about by the human action of, or toward, an individual, and by the passage of time. Further, the power of time acts differently on males and females: both have horoscopes read at birth, but girls have a second reading at menarche.[17]

Immediately after menarche occurs an astrologer is consulted and the auspicious time for the purifying bath and ceremony ascertained. The horoscope for the girl's future is worked out by confirmation of the exact

---

15   Keshini, 12, Sri Lanka 1969.
16   Steven Kemper, 'Time, person, and gender in Sinhalese astrology', *American Ethnologist*, vol. 7, no. 4, 1980, p. 745. See also Heinz Bechert, 'Remarks on astrological Sanskrit literature from Sri Lanka', in *Senarat Paranavitana Commemoration Volume, vol. 7*, Leelananda Prematilleke, Karthigesu Indrapala and J. E. van Lohuizen-de Leeuw (eds), composed by Sri Lanka Press, Leiden, The Netherlands, 1978, p. 46.
17   Kemper (1980), pp. 744, 746–747, 751.

time blood was seen. This second horoscope pertains to marriage and, according to Kemper, indicates the junction between Sinhalese culture and astrology in the concern with women's blood and impurity. The *koṭahaluva*, or menarche ceremony, links the first menstrual period with future bleeding at defloration and childbirth, and is the reason for seeking more information about the menarcheal girl through a second horoscope reading. Kemper concludes that women, as individuals, are creatures of calendar time, their stability in a marriage role being influenced by astrological lunar change. As a result, the girl at menarche is the primary focus for premarital astrology to identify her place of existence in time.[18]

In chapter three we saw that physical separation of a girl at menarche took place because of belief in *killa*, the polluting power accompanying menarche that threatens family members, particularly the men. We also saw how Keshini was immediately separated from the male members of her family by seclusion, and how the clothes and jewellery she was wearing at the onset of menarche were given to the woman who bathed her, the washing woman known as the dhobi. The dhobi, known also as *redi nändā*, is one of the key participants in the menarche ceremony. But who is the dhobi and why would she risk her own well-being by exposure to the *killa* power of the menarcheal girl, either directly in bathing her, or indirectly through handling her clothing and jewellery?[19] Winslow notes that the dhobi is one of a caste of washer-people whose duty is dirt removal, both symbolic and actual. The pure and white cloths she provides for covering the menarcheal girl are both practical and symbolic of her work. In discussion with a dhobi Winslow heard how this woman left home in the morning before her family could see her and bathed prior to returning at night. Paradoxically, although the dhobi and her family were endangered by the contagion of *killa* encountered in her work, and not negated by caste, she was equally endangered should she refuse to participate in the ritual bathing, an action which might cause her to become ill due to malevolent spirits. As compensation for her sacrifice the dhobi is paid in the gifts of personal items worn by the girl at the onset of menarche, money from the family and food prepared for the ceremony. After completing her part in the menarche ceremony, and before leaving, the dhobi blesses and forgives the girl for the dangers she has caused to her.[20] Anthropologist Karin Kapadia, writing on menarche ceremonies in rural

---

18   Kemper (1980), pp. 747–748.
19   Swarna Wickremeratne, *Buddha in Sri Lanka: Remembered Yesterdays,* State University of New York Press, Albany 2006, pp. 79–80.
20   Winslow (1980), p. 622 f.n. 13.

south India, makes two points that are relevant to Sri Lanka. One is that a dhobi can be considered as a ritual specialist. The second is that the used, but clean, clothes she brings to the newly menarcheal girl have belonged to other menarcheal girls and wearing them enhances a sense of ambiguity of identity: the identity of the child is lost and the new self not yet defined.[21]

At the end of her seclusion and as the prelude to the actual ceremony, at a time set by the astrologer, Keshini was ritually bathed once more, remembering 'at this special time the dhobi woman as well as my father's sister, that's my auntie, but it has to not be my mother's side, my father's sister helped her shower me in a separate covered place and give clothes to change. The first clothes I'm wearing are white, and [they] cover me with another white cloth, and that is how I am brought into the house. The day you come out you are still covered and you have to bring a lighted lamp. It's a brass special kind of lamp. I carried a lamp and a glass of water with the flower ... and that's why I think you have to take your shower outside somewhere because you have to come in the front door. They took me out from the back door but you are coming in the front door but you are still fully covered. I wore white, a school uniform actually. In Sri Lanka it's white. I wore a brand new school uniform covered with another white big cloth. Dhobi brought that, and I carried the lamp. You give light to the house – it's significant – but still I was fully covered, and then the dhobi breaks a coconut before I step into the house'. When asked the significance of breaking the coconut Keshini replied 'to destroy any evilness or whatever. I think that's the idea, and when they break the coconut they are expected to go like this [indicating a clean break] and be full of water. That's kind of a prosperity ... but if it goes [indicating difficulty in opening] they believe the future's not very good'. At this point in the interview we were briefly interrupted by Keshini's daughter, a university student. Keshini introduced me. 'This is my daughter. I did it for her as well even after so many years'. As my focus was on interviewing Keshini this information was a distraction and the subject was not pursued. Her daughter left and Keshini continued, 'then I came in and all my aunties, uncles, and everyone from my close family gave presents to me, gold, jewellery, earrings. I had to kneel down and worship all my relatives when they gave me presents. It is something rather special but in those days I never thought these things have meanings but any child, poor or rich, got new nice, beautiful dress ... we don't have very much ... but it's

---

21   Karin Kapadia, *Siva and her Sisters: Gender, Caste, and Class in Rural South India*, Westview Press, Boulder Colorado, 1995, p. 99.

a nice beautiful dress and the colour of the dress is also decided by whoever is doing this astrological thing ... so, that's how it is. When I was doing the same thing for my daughter I was trying to give a meaning for that'.[22]

We see from Keshini's account that her memories are mixed, partly those of a 12-year-old, and partly reflecting her re-interpretation of the long past event, but carrying the reminder of danger in this vulnerable time of transition. Change is symbolised by the identity of the women who gave Keshini the ceremonial bath – not her mother but the dhobi and Keshini's father's sisters or mother's brother's wife. Winslow points out that in the Buddhist tradition these women are classificatory mothers-in-law and suggests that their presence presages the menarcheal girl being transferred to the domination of her future mother-in-law.[23] The covering provided by the dhobi, worn over the new clothes, and the glass of water she carried protected Keshini from evil spirits, known as *vas*, as she walked with the dhobi from her bathing place to the front door. Keshini believed the breaking of the coconut destroyed any evil at the door and certainly the water might well repel *vas* but in her interviews with Buddhist Sri Lankan women, Winslow found that breaking the coconut had symbolism pertaining to domestic life, the time of marriage and a forecast of whom the dominant marriage partner would be. In her memoirs of menarche, Swarna Wickremeratne, a Buddhist woman, recalled battling to break her own coconut, the number of pieces representing the number and sex of her future children, and how the lighted lamp illuminated the wealth of food on the table, but Winslow's interviewee made no reference to any specific symbolism, so Keshini's belief in bringing light to the home is appropriate.[24]

By contrast, Nila had difficulty remembering the time frame between seclusion and ceremony but recalled she did not go back to school until the ceremony had been completed. 'I'm sort of saying that the days are fifteen or thirty, I'm not sure, but the celebration was definitely there. What happens is, that particular morning you have a bath, which three ladies gave me. All the clothes I was wearing went to a person we call dhobi. He's the washing man, or woman, who is doing our regular clothes washing, because in Sri Lanka we have someone particularly coming and washing our clothes. So

---

22 Keshini, 12, Sri Lanka 1969.
23 Winslow, (1980), pp. 606, 614. Cross-cousin marriage in a matrilineal descent system is marriage to mother's brother's son in a line where the descent is traced through the females although the power is usually is held by men. See Charlotte Seymour-Smith, *Macmillan Dictionary of Anthropology*, (1986), The Macmillan Press, London, 1993, p. 185.
24 Wickremeratne (2006), p. 80, Winslow (1980), p. 608.

he takes all those clothes he knows we will never wear again. But in the ceremony we don't have that special bath. Because I was a small-made person I didn't want to wear a sari, which is a traditional dress, but I wore a skirt and a blouse and something to cover all which is called a half-sari because that's what signifies that you've become a big girl, that you've become a woman, and you are dressed almost like a bride and everybody comes and blesses you with sandalwood, flowers, you know, like rice, they put it all on your body. Being the only girl, it was done like a party. They all bless you, give you presents and everything, but mainly this thing is done by the women. All the relatives and friends come for this thing, and my uncles gave gold coins, or something in gold as a gift, and I think now I understand the reason for that. These gold coins from every uncle they gave me as a start. I think it's to do with marriage. I think it's just an announcement that my daughter is available, but that's what I am thought to be, a big girl and available for marriage in the community or something like that, and then the ceremony as such'.

Nila continued, 'the uncle, mother's brother, is also a significant character for this blessing because I think in those days there was marriage if you had an uncle and uncle's son, you are eligible to marry. I think that could have been the reason that uncle was very prominent and they are supposed to bring dowry or something, but they don't really bring that. What they bring is their visit from their family is very important and that's the uncle that comes with his family so he brings a lot of things like clothes, flowers and things in trays, flowers and fruit and things like that and he even plays a prominent role and he puts a garland on you. You fall down and get blessing from your parents, your uncles and all the elderly people. That was very significant to us. Then people enjoy eating a meal and then after that meal you're supposed to leave for school or wherever'.[25]

The form of the menarche ceremony for Keshini and Nila follows no authoritative text but is structured by the women in the family, particularly older women, within a framework of knowledge, time and money.[26] Although the two memories of their ceremonies differ, taken together they construct a more comprehensive description of their experience. Keshini remembered seclusion, not with a sense of danger but as a place of transformation from which she would emerge as a 'blossomed flower' four weeks later. Comments on physical beauty after seclusion are not uncommon. No reference is made

---

25   Nila, 13, Sri Lanka 1964.
26   Winslow (1980), p. 607.

to her place of seclusion as being a *koṭahala gedara*, or puberty house, with its special features; rather it was 'a room' but not 'my room'. On a more reflective note, Keshini understands this seclusion to be a time of learning, of developing self-awareness, of becoming ready to enter a more 'grown up' world. Then, the astrologer is consulted and arrangements are made for her ceremony. This horoscope process is a ritual of remembering and recreation by the girl's mother, according to Winslow, although Keshini recalled it as a trendy Hindu tradition, taken up by Buddhists and part of Sri Lankan culture.[27]

Hindu Nila's ceremony, as she remembered it, commenced with a seven-day seclusion at home, in a state of transition until her ceremony 15 or 30 days later. Her one ritual bath was given on the first day of menarche by her grandmother and aunties, and we are not informed whether they were maternal or paternal. Although Nila was prohibited from seeing her father, indicating an awareness of *killa*, it was not referred to, nor was there any dhobi participation, other than taking the clothing worn at menarche, because of the dhobi's male gender. Rather, Nila's changed status as a woman was symbolised by new clothes, including the wearing of a half-sari, and celebrated with the same symbols as a Hindu bride – by the application of sandalwood, flowers and rice to her body. The menarche ceremony anticipated Nila's marriage through the presence of her maternal uncle, a dowry of gold coins and her stated eligibility to wed her uncle's son in the preferred Hindu custom of cross-cousin marriage. This signified the primacy of protection of family purity and the prevention of status ambiguity that female sexual activity outside marriage can create.[28]

The Indian interviewees emphasised that ceremony for menarche was not nation-wide in this country of many ethnic and cultural groups. Hetal from one of the hill stations of the north told me that the ceremony was specific to the southern regions. This was confirmed later by Saha: 'I'm a Hindu lady and we didn't have any ceremony. It's the south Indians who do too much fuss about it'. Alisha, from Madras, spoke briefly and indirectly of the ceremony following menarche. 'After three days they bathe. For three days, no bathing. After that they say woman can bathe. She'll be put there and all the women come and put different coloured water and things like that. Then the priest will come and a blessing will be done. Purification for the first

---

27   Winslow (1980), pp. 607, 610. See also Nisha's account in Cathryn Britton, 'Learning about "The Curse": an anthropological perspective on experiences of menstruation', *Women's Studies International Forum*, vol. 19, no. 6, 1996, pp. 650–651.
28   Winslow (1980), p. 606; Kapadia (1995), p. 104.

period takes a long time and they have to spend quite a lot of money on that'. Alisha abbreviates a menarcheal ceremony without identifying the cultural group in which it took place. The prohibition on bathing suggests a ceremony for a Brahmin caste Hindu girl, although a protracted purification ritual differs from the modern Brahmin ceremony described by Kapadia. In her comparison with that of a non-Brahmin, both taking place in Tamilnadu, in rural southern India, Kapadia arguing that change in child-marriage laws caused loss of ceremonial importance to Brahmins.[29]

Unlike the elaborate non-Brahmin puberty ceremonies, those for Brahmin girls are influenced by the belief that the reproductive role of women is secondary to that of men, Kapadia contends.[30] Women are merely vessels for the male's child. Nor do Brahmins believe that astrology indicating bad menstrual stars can affect the entire family if not ritually removed. At the onset of menarche the young girl is secluded in an area of the house, and on the fourth day the married women invited to attend the ceremony will arrive. At this juncture a Brahmin priest may become involved; otherwise married women known as *sumangali*, who are considered to be auspicious, will conduct the ceremony. Because of her impurity the menarcheal girl remains in a clearly demarcated outdoor area, indicated by a chalk design on the back porch or somewhere exterior to the house. When everyone has assembled she is called forward and seated on a low stool placed in the centre of the design. While the women sing auspicious songs one will apply auspicious substances to the girl's body, beginning with a dot of turmeric powder mixed with sesame oil on the girl's forehead and then applied to her cheeks, hands, and feet. Sesame oil is rubbed into her hair. Then one of her female relatives circles three times around the girl with a container of red *aratti* liquid, to which grains of raw rice are added, to remove any inauspiciousness. Then the container of *aratti* is carried through the house to be poured into the centre of the auspicious chalk design external to the front door. This destroys evil spirits known as *dirushti*. The menarche purification bath is given by one of the married women, whose sacrifice requires her own purifying head-bath later to leave behind all inauspiciousness and impurity, which are especially linked to the hair. After that, dressed in a new half-sari, her body and hair decorated with flowers, the young girl is incorporated into life as a young woman.[31]

29 Kapadia (1995), p. 93.
30 Kapadia (1995), p. 115.
31 Kapadia (1995), pp. 102, 108–109, 115–117.

Flowers feature very prominently in the small ceremony in Java recalled by Rara at the time of menarche (to be followed by an early marriage arranged by her grandmother). Of her menarche Rara recalled 'a day only in the pant you know? My grandmother, old woman, not tell anything, but next day my grandma gave me medicine … I don't know medicine but it was served with flower, you know, and after give me bath with flowers in the water, rose (*kanauga*), magnolia (*kautal*) and jasmine'.[32] I asked Rara if this was a Hindu tradition. 'I don't know … it might be superstitious medicine … it might be Javanese culture … and the medicine too … not in the glass but in a bowl of coconut shell with a flower too … special flower, *kautal*'. Asked if she was given new clothes to wear after her bath, Rara responded, 'yes, yes, everything new'. And the clothes worn at the onset of menarche? 'My grandma wash', indicating any power attributed to menarcheal blood was not contagious to the grandmother. Rara's ritual bath was attended by one other person. 'Another lady came making medicine for me. It's special medicine … flowers but I don't know. I think this friend from the grandmother was smart with traditional medicine. Also, I still remember when I little girl I look in the special room they got small packet for medicine … many come, you know? Small room … in her home. Very close to my grandmother … maybe my grandmother tell her … and she make for me'.

In form, Rara's menarche ceremony in Jogjakarta seems rather perfunctory. The ritual bath, given after the brief menarcheal bleeding ceased, was marked as something special only through the addition of flower petals, and Rara insisted the petals were taken from seven types of flowers although the women collectively could name only three, omitting the ubiquitous frangipani. Their symbolism remains a mystery, although Clifford Geertz, in his study of Balinese symbolism, observed that under such symbolic forms the world of the imagination and the world of ritual fuse and become the same world in which transformation of an individual's beliefs becomes possible.[33] Rara explained 'my mother and grandmother think superstitious … belief in spirit but my grandma believe in God too … is mixed … abangan'. There was no overt reference to danger, either to herself or to others, caused by her menarche and Rara reflected with some uncertainty, 'I don't know why they gave me a bath'. As there is so little written on puberty ceremonies among Javanese I have made certain extrapolations. The first is the special medicine, or *jamu*, which comes in many variations appropriate to need and

---

32   Rara, 12, Indonesia 1951.
33   Clifford Geertz, *The Interpretation of Cultures*, Basic Books, New York, 1973, p. 112.

is widely used in Indonesia, particularly in Java.[34] One concoction ensures good menstrual flow and is sold by traditional healers or by *jamu*-sellers in the markets.[35] The ingredients are classified as 'hot' and may include, for example, vinegar, yeast and ginger.[36] However, Nirmala, also from Jogjakata, remembered 'when we finish period we always have to drink *jamu*, what we call *jamu*, a herbal medicine to drink so it cleanse'.[37] Thus it would appear that Rara's *jamu* in its flower-decorated coconut shell was intended as an auspicious drink to purify the body internally after the brief menarche, rather than to ensure increased menstrual flow, with the bath providing purification compatible with religious belief within Hinduism, Islam and the animist belief in spirits.

The belief that a menarcheal girl is vulnerable to malevolent spirits belongs to an older religious belief system than the 19th-century Christian missionary overlay in the South Pacific islands, which include Fiji, home to Levani. She had not had a menarche ceremony of her own but had witnessed her older sister's, who would have an arranged marriage with a cousin to strengthen the *va-kawa*, or family ties. 'I was very young but I remember a few things that later on told me "ah, this is because she was having her period" because suddenly, just on one day, uncles started coming bringing food and I didn't know what was going on ... I think I'd have been about eight or nine and these uncles started bringing material and the mats, and aunties, and on that day my sister came dressed in traditional things and nobody told me anything and I didn't ask any questions. It was later, I think actually when I learned about culture at school which in form IV, which was when I had my period, it was when all these things came together for me ... this sister and I are very close ... and I didn't ask her ... it just didn't occur to me to ask these questions but what happened was she came out dressed in traditional clothes and there was the ceremonial thing and the *cobu* [shows clapping] and all of those things, and I remember her sitting there with her head down and then after that she went and changed and there was the

---

34 Wendy Bone, 'The magic 'Jamu'', part 1, *The Jakarta Post*, 26 July 2009.

35 Terence H. Hull and Valerie J. Hull, 'Means, motives and menses: use of herbal emmenagogues in Indonesia', in *Regulating Menstruation: Beliefs, Practices and Interpretations*, Etienne van de Walle and Elisha P. Renne (eds), University of Chicago Press, Chicago 2001, pp. 202–203.

36 Anke Niehof, 'Traditional medicine at pregnancy and childbirth in Madura, Indonesia' in *The Context of Medicines in Developing Countries: Studies in Pharmaceutical Anthropology*, Sjaak van der Geest and Susan Reynolds Whyte (eds), Kluwer Academic Publishers, Dordrecht, The Netherlands 1988, p. 240.

37 Nirmala, 13, Indonesia 1964.

feasting. She disappeared and what happened when she disappeared I don't know … whether there were other things happening and I was too young to know …. and then she appeared in these new clothes and then the feasting began … so I think … because we have the … you know, with the new baby, they have the bath and a new anointing of a chief they have the bath. A lot of the things they have the bath … and men, when they are circumcised … and I know all about that because that was open but nobody said anything and I didn't ask. I didn't even wonder what this was all about until I was in the culture class and then realised that that was her fourth day of the menarche so someone has been keeping count, but it's interesting too that my uncles and aunties came … they knew what that was for but just nobody talked about it … so in my mind I just put together that this must have been her fourth day and then I remember afterwards thinking "but it doesn't stop on the fourth day" but that's the celebration thing'.[38]

Levani's memories corroborate the findings of anthropologist Marijke Sniekers, who studied gender identity among Fijian women, including the role of the menarche ceremony.[39] Levani's sister was the first of three daughters in a family of nine children belonging to a village chief. Her menarche ceremony provided the opportunity for a major village event, one that was not repeated for the other daughters, but which anthropologists Karen Ericksen Paige and Jeffery Paige maintain provided the occasion for competitive feast-giving for a man of influence and prestige.[40] This was not an unusual situation, as Sniekers learned from her informants. Some of them believed all daughters would have menarche ceremonies, but others argued that economics determined the decision. By comparison, anthropologist Thomas Maschio found that among the Melanesian Rauto people of New Britain, the menarche ceremony was held for the eldest daughter, or for the daughter who had the most potential to become an important woman in the community, acting as a social marker for her family and giving older women an opportunity to share their knowledge and draw the young girl into their declared patterns of female social and cultural identity.[41] However, for the young Fijian girl, recognition of her menarche is the first of the steps that

---

38 Levani, 16, Fiji 1967.
39 Marijke Sniekers, 'From little girl to young woman: the menarche ceremony in Fiji', *Fijian Studies*, vol. 3, no. 2, 2005.
40 Karen Ericksen Paige and Jeffery M. Paige, *The Politics of Reproductive Ritual*, University of California Press, Berkeley, 1982, p. 52.
41 Thomas Maschio, 'Mythic images and objects of myth in Rauto female puberty ritual', in *Gender Rituals: Female Initiation in Melanesia*, Nancy C. Lutkehaus and Paul B. Roscoe (eds), Routledge, New York, 1995, p. 136.

will take her to identifying herself as a woman. She tells someone, and if it is her aunt or a friend the news will be conveyed to her mother, hence to her father. The form of the ceremony begins with a four-day seclusion inside the house, during which time the women of her family, her grandmother, mother, aunts, and cousins if she is from a chiefly family, begin the instruction that van Gennep refers to as the liminal rites of transition, when the specific knowledge of women is shared with her. She learns about menstruation and menstrual hygiene, female sexuality and the importance to her family of her virginity at marriage, motherhood and the social meanings attached to being a woman in her society, including behavioural warnings, narrated through stories, myth and family history.[42]

During this time invitations are sent out by her father, inviting close and extended family to his daughter's menarche ceremony. Because Levani's sister was from a chiefly family, invitations would go to the *mataqali*, those from other villages who are part of the chiefdom. Some family members arrive during the four-day seclusion to enable the women to share in the young girl's transition. Everyone brings gifts of food, the decorated bark cloth known as *tapa*, and mats called *masi*, which have great ceremonial and practical value. Most significantly they greet the young girl as a member of their adult community. Inside the house the young girl is cared for by her female relatives. She is washed, dressed and fed while sitting, resting or sleeping on a pile of mats, her movements restricted to toilet visits or brief walks for the four days of seclusion. Bathing, and swimming in the sea or the river during this time, is prohibited, as is going outside the house, because the power of menarcheal blood may harm others, and the evil spirits outside may harm the young girl or her women companions during this vulnerable transition state. Levani referred to the four days as 'a celebration thing' which Sniekers' informants verified. Fijian celebration and ceremony for birth, marital consummation, and mourning are all four days according to ancestral tradition.[43]

Levani remembered her sister's reappearance in traditional dress on the fourth night, her coming out. In preparation the young girl would be bathed and her body rubbed with coconut oil so her skin gleamed. She wore the distinctive traditional *masi* dress with a *salusalu* or sweetly fragrant flower garland, and stepped over the threshold to become the centre of attention, seated in the usual position of the chief at the head of the eating mat, the chief

---

42   Sniekers (2005), pp. 405, 406–407. See also van Gennep trans. Vizedom and Caffee (1960), p. 11.

43   Sniekers (2005), pp. 406–407, 409–410, 412.

and elders beside her, receiving more gifts of masi and mats known as yau, or wealth, in a formal ceremony associated with the *cobu* or hand-clapping that Levani had recalled. After the ceremony, these gifts are redistributed among the relatives, except for the mats and *masi* touched by her menarcheal body during her seclusion, and personal items. Then Levani's sister disappeared briefly to change her clothes, her new status publicly symbolised by the long wrap-around skirt or *sulu* and by her distinctive round haircut. On her return prayers for the young girl were said, the food was blessed and the feast began, with the young girl being offered the choicest bits. Speeches were given, her father's acknowledging that his daughter was now a woman. Sniekers considers that change in her collective identity is symbolised by her position in the adult group where she faces the men as a woman, and faces the children as an adult. Her individual identity continues to transform as she assumes more adult responsibility, learning slowly the lessons taught by her female kin during her four-day menarcheal ceremony.[44] Those four days are not all that's required to become a woman, but rather, as anthropologist Nancy Lutkehaus argues in her work among Melanesian societies of the South Pacific, it is but one of the rituals that a woman participates in that incrementally forms her gender identity and full 'personhood' in a particular society.[45]

As societies undergo change so, too, do their ceremonies. Menarche ceremonies in Fiji are one example. Before 19th-century Christian missionaries began their conversion process in the Fijian Islands, and compulsory education took girls away from home, the feast at the end of the menarche ceremony was followed by the commencement of intricate tattooing that visibly and permanently marked the young girl as a woman. This slow and painful process required breaks for the skin to heal and the throbbing to settle and, when completed, the girl's lower body was covered from waist to knee, resembling a pair of bike shorts. Four nights later another ceremony took place in which a feast, given by the family of the girl's promised husband, placed the young girl once more at the centre of attention, proud of her endurance that signified her to be a brave woman and permitted to wear a *liku*, or skirt made of fibre. Missionary influence led to cessation of this part of the menarche ritual.[46] In neighbouring Tonga the menarche ceremony

---

44   Sniekers (2005), pp. 413–415.
45   Nancy C. Lutkehaus, 'Feminist anthropology and female initiation in Melanesia', in *Gender Rituals: Female Initiation in Melanesia,* Nancy C. Lutkehaus and Paul B. Roscoe (eds), Routledge, New York 1995, p. 13.
46   Sniekers (2005), p. 416–419.

for girls has not been recorded since the 1930s, according to anthropologist Helen Morton, and tattooing was prohibited by 19th-century missionaries who considered it to be a 'heathen practice'.[47]

We have seen certain commonalities in the form and symbolism of the menarche ceremonies described by the interviewees and interpreted through secondary scholarship. The body of the menarcheal girl may be likened to a chrysalis or budding flower but is more complex because of the ambiguous connotation with power and vulnerability, hence seclusion during this transitional or liminal state. In certain situations an individual, designated by caste, makes a symbolic sacrifice of themselves by acceptance of the menarcheal girl's clothing, which contains the pollutive power of menarcheal blood, and by accepting the possibility of pollution through contact with water from the body of the menarcheal girl during the ritual bathing. In seclusion the girl is not left alone because of her vulnerability to malevolent spirits. Her most significant companions are the older women of her family, the grandmothers and aunts, who symbolise the knowledge of all women, expressed through stories that tell of strength and endurance, of sexuality and reproduction, and of protective and nurturing maternal skills, intended to mould and shape the changing identity of the young girl to young woman. Common to all ceremonies is the ritual bath symbolising purity, and new clothes symbolising the change in social status when incorporated into adult society.

Each of the women interviewed remembered their ceremony, or that of their older sister, but their recollection was overlaid by their interpretation of the events they were retelling. There was some confusion over time and sequence of events, and focus varied between loss – of personal items to the dhobi – and gain – gifts received or new clothes. The symbolism of ceremonial artefacts, lamps, flowers, coverings and medicine were not fully understood at the time and interestingly, as an educated adult Keshini sought meaning in her menarche ceremony through that of her Australian-born daughter. Although her disengagement from her ceremony in the re-telling, indicated by the use of the impersonal 'they' rather than the collective 'we', suggested cynicism, perhaps for my benefit, Keshini would not imperil her daughter by ignoring Buddhist belief in *killa*, and ensured a menarche ceremony was given. I didn't pursue details because the age and birthplace of the daughter did not fit interview requisites. Levani recalled her sister 'sitting there with her head down', represented more as a ceremonial object than as subject and,

---

47   Helen Morton, *Becoming Tongan: an Ethnography of Childhood,* University of Hawai'i Press, Honolulu 1996, pp. 113–114.

given that their father was the village chief, the ceremonial feast-giving placed him in the central role. This leads to asking how others might benefit from a menarche ceremony. For the older female relatives who are with the girl through her seclusion there are opportunities for strengthening family ties; historically for Indian Hindus the family benefited economically once their marriage dowry was completed and their daughter was transferred to her husband. In more recent times, as Nila remarked, the menarche ceremony has social benefits by allowing parents to make 'an announcement that my daughter is … available'.

Although this collection of stories is limited, one conclusion seems clear. A menarche ceremony is not solely for the benefit of the girl whose experience it is. The cultures who maintain the ceremony in some form, based on blood pollution and danger, provide evidence that a woman remains subject to men, both father and husband, and that this social condition is perpetuated by older married women in the passing of knowledge during the transformative or liminal time of seclusion. Through van Gennep's tripartite framework we are able to understand that there are more similarities than differences in menarche ceremonies. Judith Brown found that the ceremony endorses the changed status of girls in communities where they remain in the maternal home after marriage, and that ceremony is more widespread in societies where women contribute significantly to subsistence activities, although the stories I was told by interviewees from cultures in the process of industrialisation, with resulting social change reflected in ceremonial traditions, have no bearing on this.

In the beginning of this chapter I suggested that we have no tradition of menarche ceremonies in Anglo-Australia. Indeed, menarche is symbolised by silence. Nonetheless, there are rite-of-passage ceremonies that take place at or around the time of menarche, allowing transition of a young person to another status recognised by their social group. I was reminded of this by Marjorie, an English-born woman, who remembered with some horror the discovery of blood 'in the evening and I was going to a church social and I was wearing my confirmation dress which was a white crepe dress'.[48] Marjorie's confirmation, her special white dress and her anticipated church social all reflect a change of status through the religious ceremony of confirmation, which admitted her to full church membership and participation in Holy Communion, followed by inclusion in church-related social activities for her peer group. As divinity professor, John Macquarrie observes:

---

48   Marjorie, 12, England 1956.

solemnity is heightened because this sacrament comes at a point of life when the recipient is leaving childhood behind and is facing the new and increasing responsibilities that will come with adult life. This is why confirmation is for many people an impressive and well-remembered moment in their lives.[49]

Marjorie was 12 years old at menarche – the usual age for confirmation – and beginning secondary school, and we will examine her experience through van Gennep's three-stage theory of ceremony: separation, transition and incorporation, which in Marjorie's life coincided with her menarche. In the articles of faith, directives for the Church of England (as the Anglican Church was then known), confirmation was considered desirable at coming of age, an opportunity for the child to ratify baptismal promises made by godparents on behalf of the infant.[50] At the time of Marjorie's confirmation, preparation involved separation from usual activities to attend special classes focusing on catechism, which is the doctrine of the church in a question–answer format, and the meaning and symbolism of the two main sacraments, baptism and Holy Communion. On the day of their confirmation young girls wore a modest white dress with a white veil covering their hair. They were separated from family and friends and seated together at the front of the church, their confirmatory vows made collectively in an atmosphere that was both restrained and serious. In front of them the confirming bishop, robed in the full regalia of office, received each individual confirmation candidate presented to him. They knelt before him to receive a blessing by prayer and the symbolic laying on of hands to the head symbolising the gift of the Holy Spirit. There usually remained an interval of some days before taking first communion, a liminal time of anticipation. At first communion the newly confirmed young girl was aware that she was now an adult member of the church and, as such, was incorporated through greetings of welcome by well-wishers.[51]

We can see, in the religious basis for confirmation, links to the medieval past when the cult of virginity, promulgated by the Catholic Church, imposed a form of control on young girls at the time of menarche through chaste

---

49   John Maquarrie, 'Confirmation', in *A Guide to the Sacraments*, Continuum, New York 1999, p. 84.
50   'Articles of religion XXV' and 'The order of confirmation' in *The Book of Common Prayer* (1662), Oxford University Press, London, n.d., c.1950, p. 433, 228.
51   'The order of confirmation' pp. 228–230 and memories of own experience in 1951. I have focused on young girl candidates although confirmation was not necessarily gender specific.

behaviour.[52] In Western Christian tradition, confirmation, established by the fourth century, symbolised religious transformation from child to responsible young adult, corresponding with a physical transformation silently signified by menarche. This increased emphasis on the spiritual contested the dangers of burgeoning sexuality and potential sexual corruption, hence the white dress and head-covering acting as both symbol and reminder of the purity already bestowed by the ritually blessed water of baptism. Whereas Roman Catholic girls were confirmed well before puberty, the Anglican and other Protestant churches had the ceremony as a recognition of coming of age.[53] Specific to Latin America, particularly Mexico, is the Roman Catholic coming-of-age ceremony for girls, which is not widely known but worth introducing. It is *la quinceañera*, argued by anthropologist Karen Mary Davalos to be a statement of gender identity and ethnicity. Preparation takes the form of special classes focusing on religious and social responsibilities, including the Catholic ideal of pre-marital sexual purity.

On the day of the quinceañera the young girl, attired in a special dress resembling a bridal gown, walks to the church in procession with her parents, godparents, and immediate family. Inside the church she renews baptismal vows, gives thanks for surviving 15 years, and prays for a strengthening of religious faith. The religious service is commonly followed by a social ceremony in the form of a big party with dancing, marking the transition from young girl to young, responsible, adult.[54] Interestingly, when asked about ceremony at time of menarche none of my Chilean interviewees made any reference to the quinceañera but all referred to the expectation of heterosexual pre-marital purity.

Nor was my Jewish contributor able to explain the experience of a bat mitzvah as circumstances prevented her from undergoing it, but the ceremony ought not to be overlooked. In the Jewish tradition a girl comes of religious age at 12 years and one day in the presence of pubertal signs.[55] Although efforts were made in the 19th and 20th centuries to recognise this

---

52 See chapter one.
53 Macquarie (1999), p. 80; Ivan G. Marcus, *The Jewish Life Cycle: Rites of Passage from Biblical to Modern Times*, University of Washington Press, Seattle 2004, p. 111. See also Mandy Ross, *Coming of Age*, Heinemann Library, Oxford 2003, pp. 6–7. This is a text for young people describing cultural rites of passage.
54 Karen Mary Davalos, 'La Quinceañera: making gender and ethnic identities', *Frontiers: A Journal of Women's Studies*, vol. 16, nos 2/3, 1996, pp. 109–111, 120–121.
55 Bloch (1980), p. 19. At the time of Sinai puberty was estimated by the growth of a minimal two pubic hairs.

coming of age in parts of Warsaw and Lemberg, now Lvov, the occasion warranted a party rather than a religious ritual in a synagogue. In parts of mid 19th-century Italy, girls and boys who had come of age were blessed by the rabbi, and recited a blessing in a ceremony marking their entry to the *minyan*, the quorum of ten, usually men, required for community prayer, public readings of the Torah, and other spiritual matters.[56] In France at the same time, Jewish confirmation with the young girl wearing the white bridal-style dress of a much younger Catholic confirmation candidate was introduced, and in Germany, the Jewish Reform Movement, influenced by Protestantism, attempted to replace the traditional bar mitzvah with a newer ceremony for 15 or 16-year-old boys and girls following religious education of some duration, including a Jewish catechism in question–answer format.[57] In the US, the first specially created ceremony, according to Jewish historian Ivan Marcus, was that of Rabbi Mordecai Kaplan for his 12-year-old daughter, Judith, in 1922.[58] Over the next three decades the ceremony of bat mitzvah took form in Conservative and Reform synagogues, integrated with the Friday night service with the young girl, given the honour of reading the *haftarah*, the writings of the prophets through whom God spoke to the Jewish people. The *haftarah* was linked with the weekly reading of the Torah, due to be recited by a man the following day.[59] Conservative synagogues introduced a confirmation ceremony for girls who attained a religious study goal in the synagogue school reflecting the Christian model, including the white dress, and often held at Shavuot, a time of spiritual redemption of the Jewish people. However it took the rise of Jewish feminism in the 1980s, with its demand for egalitarian liturgical involvement, to slowly evolve bat mitzvah to a Sabbath ceremony in progressive synagogues, in which a 13-year-old girl would read from the Torah, ask blessings over the Torah, read *haftarah* and make a speech to the congregation in the same way as boys at their bar mitzvah. Resistance to change from Orthodox Judaism has brought about innovative shifts in Jewish feminist thought, including services specifically for women to counter the non-acceptance of egalitarian ritual in mixed services, which, among other issues, is partly based on the dignity of the congregation

---

56 Marcus (2004), pp. 105–106. For an explanation of Jewish terms see 'Judaism 101: a glossary of basic Jewish terms, concepts and practices', a project of the Union of Orthodox Jewish Congregations of America, http://www.ou.org
57 Marcus (2004), p. 113. See also Bloch (1980), p. 22.
58 Marcus (2004), pp. 106–107.
59 Marcus (2004), p. 109.

and the historic belief that a woman reading the Torah indicates that men in the community are unlearned. Other services, apart from the regular, are attended by groups of Orthodox Jews and permit certain liturgical participation of women. There is some inclusion of girls who have reached twelve to read the Torah and to receive *'aliyot*, the call to read the Torah, although the ceremony of bat mitzvah appears to remain a troubled work-in-progress for mixed Sabbath congregations.[60]

Memorising a sacred text is part of the rite of passage ending in ceremony for young Muslim boys and girls, but one that none of my Arabic speakers from Lebanon made reference to. Known as the *Khatum Qur'an*, also called the Muslim Hatum Ceremony, it takes place when the young person is between the ages of 10 and 12 years, that is about the time of a girl's menarche. It is a slow and disciplined endeavour beginning at about five to seven years of age under the supervision of a Qur'an teacher, with the intention to read correctly, and to understand, the entire Qur'an. In Malaysia the ceremony was part of the Islamic revival of the 1980s, enabling the young girl who succeeds to be commended by her teacher, bring pride to her family, and achieve the special community status of being a good Muslim who knows the Qur'an. To mark her change in status, a special all-female ceremony and feast are held and at this ceremony the young girl completes her reading. She is dressed in white, indicating purity, and behaves with appropriate decorum. In a ceremony-within-the-ceremony, the women guests sing the *marhaban*, or praise to Allah, while the hosts of the ceremony distribute *bunga telur*, or egg flowers, and sprinkle *minyak attah*, an Arabian perfume, on the singing women, as a way of thanking them for their attendance and for witnessing the completed reading of the Qur'an.[61]

The support of women at this transitional time of a young girl's life is present in a peculiarly social ceremony with historical economic symbolism: the debutante ball. It is a ceremony that Karen Ericksen Paige finds not unlike menarcheal ceremonies in traditional cultures, arguing that the American debutante ball is a display of paternal wealth and prestige advertising a daughter's worth to prospective suitors, who are expected to

---

60   Marcus (2004), pp. 110, 114–116. See also Elana Sztokman, 'Some rabbinic sources on women and Torah reading', compiled in honour of her daughter Avigayil's bat-mitzvah, 22 January 2005, p. 3. http://www.shira.org.au/learn/read/
61   Nor Faridah Abdul Manaf, 'Other coming of age rituals among Malay Muslim girls in Malaysia', in *The Encyclopedia of Women and Islamic Cultures: Family, Body, Sexuality and Health, Vol. 3*, Suad Joseph and Afsaneh Najmabadi (eds), Koninklijke Brill NV, Leiden, The Netherlands, 2006, pp. 69–70. See also Ross (2003), pp. 10–11.

be drawn from the same social class the ball indicates she will be part of.[62] Sociologist Dean Knudsen attributes the ceremony to European courts of the 17th century, but historians Isobel Thompson and Vicki Northey focus on England, arguing that the debutante ball is a Victorian upper-class tradition that introduced a young woman to adult social life through presentation at court, followed by a flurry of social activities through the spring and summer seasons. However, Australian social researcher Lyn Harrison found that by the late 1960s, the effects of social change had significantly reduced the popularity of the debutante ball.[63] Historian Janet McCalman's research, comparing the experiences of middle-class Melbourne girls from two private girls' schools, provided evidence that the debutante ball waned in popularity after the Second World War with formal debuts at Genazzano, a Catholic school, being 48 per cent, and at Methodist Ladies College, where many thought it 'corny', only 24 per cent.[64]

How corny would these girls have found the concept of an initiation cere-mony? Van Gennep described the time as social rather than physical puberty and theorised that the initiation ceremony took the young person from the world of the asexual to that of the sexual. Such ceremonies made the girl marriageable, and was that not the original intention of the debutante ball?[65] Following van Gennep's framework of separation, transition and incorporation, the young potential debutante, past menarche but at the age of increasing independence and assuming some responsibility for herself, enters a time of training under the guidance of an experienced woman in preparation for presentation to a figure of some community standing. She learns good posture, how to move gracefully in a long dress and how to curtsy – left foot forward and right foot behind, bending with straight back – while extending the right hand.[66] In her study of constructions of femininity through the debutante ball, Harrison found that young women

---

62 Karen Ericksen Paige, 'Social aspects of menstruation', in *Cultural Perspectives on Biological Knowledge*, Troy Duster and Karen Garrett (eds), Ablex Publishing Company, New Jersey, 1984, p. 139.

63 Dean D. Knudsen, 'Socialization to elitism: a study of debutantes', *The Sociological Quarterly*, vol. 9, no. 3, 1968, p. 300. Isobel Thompson and Vicki Northey, *Coming Out: Debutante Balls*, Wangaratta Travelling Exhibition curated by Albury Regional Museum and The Exhibitions Gallery, 1991, p. 3 cited in Lyn Harrison, "It's a nice day for a white wedding': the debutante ball and constructions of femininity', *Feminism and Psychology*, vol. 6, no. 4, 1997, pp. 497–498.

64 Janet McCalman, *Journeyings: The Biography of a Middle-Class Generation 1920–1990*, (1993), Melbourne University Press, Carlton 1995, p.189 and f.n. 14, p. 189.

65 Van Gennep trans. Vizedom and Caffee (1960), pp. 65–68.

66 'Coming out, ready or not', *Sydney Morning Herald*, 30 November 2004.

in their final year of secondary school in a regional Victorian city enjoyed creating themselves as debutantes. Their separation and preparation included dancing lessons and carefully planning a romanticised feminine appearance as a modest, marriageable virgin, symbolised by a long white dress with elbow-length gloves, representing purity.[67] The ceremony focused on the debutante, her male partner taking only a supporting role, in a night of evanescent transformation. Although the young women knew that the debutante ball resembled a wedding, they didn't think the historic purpose of the occasion had any relevance to them. The ceremony allowed them a time of liminality, pleasure and creativity, summed up by Harrison as filling a niche that allows these young women to feel special, living out a fantasy of doing something a little bit better than anyone else, and helping in the construction of identity. Yet the process of incorporation fails at community level, affecting only the individual who may say with some pride, 'look at me, I'm part of society', without society recognising or valuing any change in her status. Debutante balls in this context fail to fulfill Schlegel and Barry III's definition of initiation ceremony.[68] Nevertheless the significance of the ceremony to the participants is clear since two years later, when each young woman was asked for the highlight of her life, she unhesitatingly replied 'the deb ball'.[69] In this regard there is considerable difference between the contemporary debutante ball in provincial Victoria and its counterpart in late 1960s US where, Knudsen argues, the purpose was less an introduction to society, which had probably been experienced for some time, and more a public transition to high-status marriageability.[70]

Conclusion

Interview findings confirmed that the cultural meanings associated with menarche were based on control of the menarcheal body and of the environment surrounding that body. The ceremonies that were described reveal a cultural belief that by intervention and ritual purification, a young girl rendered vulnerable by menarche would be protected from the dangers of possession. In recalling their experiences, women remembered the early stage of separation more acutely, and interpreted it at varying levels of significance, according to their youthful perception and focus at the time.

---

67   Harrison, (1997), pp. 496, 505.
68   Schlegel and Barry III (1979), p. 199.
69   Harrison (1997), pp. 504, 507, 509.
70   Knudsen (1968), p. 301.

We saw the contrast between the loss expressed by Keshini and the gain expressed by Nila, but whether the symbolism invoked by material objects translated to the loss and gain of identity, or to the power and vulnerability of the menarcheal body is doubtful. We saw that certain symbols are common to all menarche ceremonies described, including water for purification, new clothes indicating new status, food shared in reciprocity for attendance, and gifts given to celebrate not just menarche but the next life event: money and gifts symbolising dowry wealth; spices and rice symbolising marriage.

One feature that was common to most of the ceremonies was the post-ceremonial mixed-gender feasting. Descriptions of it indicated the reproductive capital brought to the family by the menarche of a daughter. In Sri Lanka this was demonstrated through the cultural custom of arranged marriage to a cross-cousin, an arrangement somewhat at odds with the return to school by the girl at the conclusion of her ceremony.

The importance of the menarche ceremony to interviewees was evident in the decisions by both Keshini and Nila to have menarche ceremonies for their Australian-born daughters. This indicated two important aspects of their lives as an immigrant woman – their belief in their daughters' vulnerability at menarche, regardless of changed geographical and cultural circumstances, and a desire to acknowledge the cultural significance of the ceremony to Sri Lankan-Australian women.

In comparison with the menarche ceremony, religious and secular ceremonies occurring at or close to menarche revealed two important differences – the absence of belief in danger caused by transitional spirit possession and the component of choice in participation. Although most of the ceremonies were individually focused, confirmation usually involved a group with an individual ritual component. Studying the core religious text at a deeper level prepared the individual for her status transition from child to adult within church, synagogue, or mosque. In close-knit community groups, acknowledgement of changed status would occur. Commonalities were present in both religious and secular ceremonies, in the ritual symbolism of dress, demeanour and the manner in which knowledge of the new status was demonstrated. Social support of the individual by family members, teachers, and friends was common to all participants; so, too, was the reciprocal strengthening of family and social ties through the sharing of food at the end of the ceremony. The anomaly was the debutante ball, a secular ceremony that fulfilled the criteria of a transitional ceremony, focusing on the presentation of young women to a prominent and usually male figure, symbolising request and acceptance into the society of adults and sexuality.

Although the secular and religious ceremonies give young women choice in participation they are nonetheless ceremonies of control, influencing the ways in which young women might live a particular religious or social life. Even so, the argued psychological benefits of secular ceremonies such as the debutante ball are worth consideration.

Chapter 5

MENSTRUAL LORE

You can't touch the trees. They will die.[1]

'You can't touch the trees. They will die'. The statement, made by the totally modern-looking woman seated opposite me, had a certain shock value in this society of advanced technology and instant communication. Yet why should I be surprised? Few women growing up in the 1950s and 1960s would be unfamiliar with these so-called old wives' tales, anecdotes of magic and women's lore, usually greeted with derision or fascination as part of an informal education beginning at menarche and centring on women's life matters. These were not stories in the sense of fairy tales but brief warnings, prescriptions or prohibitions that might be embroidered to make a point, shared between mother and daughter or friends who heard them from older female relatives. Some were believable and others frankly bizarre. Rosalia first heard about the power of menstrual blood when she experienced menarche in Sicily. Later, having migrated to Australia to settle in Melbourne, she recalled 'we used to have a lemon tree with lemons all year round. You know what? One person went there and she loved lemons and she picked the lemons and she said it was so beautiful. Whether she had her period or not – from then on the tree went backwards'.[2]

Was this menstrual magic or a way of explaining the inexplicable? And ought we to be surprised to learn that the same belief remains part of cultural life for some young immigrant girls in Melbourne?[3] These cautionary stories or anecdotes had a very real place in the life of girls at menarche in the recent past, and many continue to be observed among certain cultural groups today. In this chapter we will explore several issues.

---

1   Maria, 14 years old at menarche, Italy 1957.
2   Rosalia, 13, Italy 1950.
3   Fida Sanjakdar, "Teacher talk': the problems, perspectives and possibilities of developing a comprehensive sexual health education curriculum for Australian Muslim students', *Sex Education*, vol. 9, no. 3, 2009, p. 267.

First, the similarities and differences between the stories recalled by women from diverse cultures. Second, the purpose served by menstrual lore and the meanings inferred by it. Third, where does the lore come from and what is the reason for its survival? Fourth, is women's menstrual lore a part of all cultural histories and what is its relevance for girls in today's societies?

The mode of transmission of women's menstrual lore reflected the oral tradition of many cultures, and the fact that, even among cultures that are gaining a literate tradition, non-literacy is still predominant among women. Menstrual lore was a blending of myth and folklore that was entirely secular. For instance, at the onset of her menarche Maria feared she was sick. Her mother reassured her of her normality, at the same time warning her 'not to use cold water. It's no good and she told me not to have vinegar and not to have a lemon with my period. I didn't know why but she explained to me it's no good for you. No good for the blood'. Maria continued 'you can't touch the trees. They will die'. She repeated this twice for emphasis, continuing 'and if we make the sauce not to touch the sauce and not to go near the sauce or the wine. Not to touch the grapes when you make wine 'cause it will go off'.[4]

The warning about the effects of vinegar and lemon juice were unfamiliar to Rosalia, in Sicily, although she had been warned about touching certain things, including tomatoes being made into sauce, remembering that 'we used to make it in a big dish and dry it out in the sun and put in a lot of salt and then you put it away. You cover it with special material ... it stays all winter. Mum said "when you've got your period don't go near", and not all women, but lot of women, have a very strong period and if they touch a plant or a tree it would have died'.[5] Rosalia introduces two important issues here. Firstly, that not all Italian women share the same menstrual folklore and, secondly, that the effect of the menstruous touch does not belong to all women but primarily to those who have greater menstrual power or strength.

Among the second group of Italian women, Loretta did not believe that the touch of a menstruating woman might kill plants, but she was definite that 'if you make a tomato sauce and you have your period the tomatoes don't come good. They go off. There they cook a lot of sauce and when you go to help they ask "do you have your period?" If you say you do they say "no, no, no you can't"'.[6] Yet not all women shared this menstrual

4   Maria, 14, Italy 1957.
5   Rosalia, 13, Italy 1950.
6   Loretta, 10, Italy 1947.

lore either. It had no part in Neve's earlier life – 'my mother not do this no touch this, no touch that'[7] – and Alcina moved from a small town to Rome shortly after menarche – 'I live in the city … and city life … I've never heard'[8] – indicating the belief may have been confined to rural areas.

But the idea of harm emanating from the menarcheal and menstruating girl was evident in many other cultures. Within the rural area of northern Uganda, tribal belief in this destructive power was transmitted to Cecile at menarche. 'They told me not to climb on the fruit trees because they will rot … like mangoes … the girls with periods are not allowed to climb the trees'.[9] She recalled that girls and women were prohibited from drinking milk when menstruating but it took further reading to discover it was because of the belief that production of milk from the cows would be affected.[10] Cecile made reference to menstrual avoidance of touching certain foods but from a practical viewpoint, 'sometimes you couldn't, but then it also depends on the women who prepare food. Even cutting a pineapple which they will do, they don't, and you wouldn't tell people [laughs] … but a woman has to cook'.

Menstrual prohibitions extended to questions about care of the menstruating woman's body, including food that was to be avoided, and sometimes the need to protect the body from water. Ramona remembered 'my mum told me I can't wash my hair … because the blood will stop and something's going to happen to you and is no good. I could have a shower but no long shower … but not to wash my hair. She told me never to go in the bath'.[11] Beatriz, also recalled her mother's instructions 'you don't wash hair … you don't eat any sour things like lemons'.[12] This was endorsed by Lola. 'I wasn't allowed to have a shower. Nothing to do with cold water because Mum said … I remember I asked why, and she said "because your

7   Neve, 11, Italy 1941.
8   Alcina, 15, Italy 1947.
9   Cecile, 16, Uganda 1965.
10   Varina Tjon A. Ten, 'Menstrual Hygiene as a big taboo', *Menstrual Hygiene: a Neglected Condition for the Achievement of Several Millennium Development Goals*, European Commission – EuropeAid, Zoetermeer, 2007, p. 6.
11   Ramona, 15, Chile 1964. Cold water avoidance, hair-washing, ice-cream and cold drink prohibition during menstruation was widely practised among certain Spanish women who experienced menarche prior to 1975, according to anthropologist Britt-Marie Thurén in 'Opening doors and getting rid of shame: experiences of first menstruation in Valencia, Spain', *Women's Studies International Forum*, vol. 17, nos. 2–3, 1994, pp. 219, 222.
12   Beatriz, 12, Chile c.1960.

period is going to stop", and not to drink lemon. I used to love lemon. I used to cut a lemon in half and eat it, licking with salt, and now she said "no. No lemon at all"'. I asked for further explanation. 'It is like a coagulant, and I think they believe that because in our country when we kill a lamb, we keep the blood. When you get the blood it's just liquid blood ... but if you put a lot of lemon in ... you're congealing it like a jelly and I think that was the belief, so if you drank lemon juice the period blood would congeal and I wasn't allowed to touch the salad with the lemon juice dressing'.[13]

The theme of water and its effect on the menstruating body was recalled widely among my interviewees. Aleli in the Philippines learned that 'when you have your period you're not to have a shower the whole week. No showers until your period finishes. There is a word in Tagalog [Filipino language] that they call "pas mal". I don't know how to translate it to English but they said if you have the shower when you have your period, when you grow older you will have pains and aches'.[14] Aleli pointed out that showers in the Philippines were never hot. Ria related similar lore. 'When you've got your period first day, second day, third day you don't bathe. That's not allowed. I don't remember why but you're not allowed to do that. Just sponge down and clean yourself ... not to get it in the vagina or even taking a shower ... but really like bathing you have to wait until the thing has gone'.[15] Corazon's cousins were her informants. Their response to her menarche was urgent: 'come, come, quick, quick, you have your shower, quick, but after this you shouldn't shower any more because when you have your period you're not allowed'.[16] Nadia, born to a Lebanese mother in Alexandria, remembered being told that 'we shouldn't wash ourselves during the period. I asked my mother why. She said "you'll have heavy bleeding because of the hot water"'.[17] For Greek girls it was swimming rather than washing that was the issue. Alexandria-born Zosime recalled 'we had showers there just boiling water in the tin and put some cold to make warm. Showers after toilet. Never be unclean',[18] and Alexandria-born Meletta, remembered 'we have showers, cold showers but only showers. We don't go to swimming'.[19] This was endorsed by Athene, whose mother told her 'you wash yourself, but

13   Lola, 17, Chile 1967.
14   Aleli, 10, Philippines 1959.
15   Ria, 13, Philippines 1955.
16   Corazon, 12, Philippines 1956.
17   Nadia, 11, Lebanon 1950.
18   Zosime, 11, Egypt 1934.
19   Meletta, 13, Egypt, year unknown.

no shower. No swimming'.[20] In the Philippines Erlinda recalled 'we're not allowed to have a shower until the third day when it's finished'.[21]

Prohibition of hair washing was widely reported. Maryam, a Christian from Lebanon, told me 'we were not allowed to wash our hair when we had a period'. I asked why and was informed 'it's to protect her health because they believe when a girl has her period all the veins and arteries would be open and the hormones different so she will be more vulnerable to infection'.[22] Maria, in Italy, also recalled being told 'I cannot wash my hair'.[23] Marjorie, in northern England, regarded it as an old wives' tale: 'you didn't wash your hair when you have a period. I don't know why but I think it was because you were considered not to be very well. And when you weren't well, when you had a cold, you didn't wash your hair because we didn't have hairdryers in those days and we had, always had long thick hair. We didn't say "she's menstruating" or "she's got a period" but "she's unwell". We certainly couldn't go swimming, and we did swimming at school, so all the girls who had their periods would sit on the bench. As far as baths go I can't remember but we only got a bath once a week'.[24] Violetta, in the Philippines, remembered being told by her grandmother and aunties 'not to take a bath but to wash in warm water ... not hair'.[25] This was corroborated by Corazon, who recalled, 'you're not allowed to have a shower, especially if you wet your head you'll go crazy'.[26]

Restrictions on the foods a menstruating girl could eat were also widespread, although in some cases the women interviewed had not experienced them directly. Aleli noted that in the Philippines 'you must not eat food that's acidic like vinegar, green mangoes, anything with acid ... sour in taste. It has to do with the passing of the blood. It will stop'.[27] Levani, in Fiji, had vague recollections of hearing about menstrual traditions but has never been instructed by women members of her family. 'I know that in other islands, Vanuatu for instance, there are certain kinds of food they are not allowed to touch while they are having their period. I don't remember anything like that in Fiji'.[28] Virisila, however, remembered 'my mum and

---

20   Athene, 13, Greece c.1956.
21   Erlinda, 12, Philippines 1964.
22   Maryam, 15, Lebanon 1942.
23   Maria, 14, Italy 1957.
24   Marjorie, 12, England 1956.
25   Violetta, 14, Philippines 1938.
26   Corazon, 12, Philippines 1956.
27   Aleli, 10, Philippines 1959.
28   Levani, 16, Fiji 1967.

my auntie mentioned that when they had their period they were told not to shower for four days, and they were supposed not to eat certain foods ... I think some kinds of leaves and some seafood. I remember asking them why that particular food and they said "we don't know. That's all we were told. We don't know why"'.[29]

Menstrual food avoidance from menarche onward was remembered by Sue, a highly educated Chinese woman who told me the 'only thing I can remember is my mother said "OK, no eating stuff like pineapple"'. It was believed that 'particular foods would coagulate the blood a bit more'. To Sue, food avoidance 'was more the kind of thing where they just said "look, it was too cooling" – the usual heating-cooling business we have in foods – "it was too cooling so stay away from that kind of thing"'.[30] Qing, also Chinese, remembered 'certain do's and don'ts when we are experiencing the menarche. They advised me not to take the cold drinks because it would increase period pain'.[31] Nirmala, in Indonesia, was told by her mother and grandmother to avoid eating egg during her period 'because it gives the blood the strong smell'.[32] Ria recalled food avoidance in the Philippines and how 'we usually eat mangoes, green mangoes, that's what we really like. We're not allowed to eat the sour thing you know? The blood doesn't flow'.[33] Violetta heard the lore from her grandmother and aunties. 'You will not eat sour fruits. They say the blood will clot'[34] and Corazon heard 'you're not allowed to have vinegar, any sour things ... green mangoes ... because your blood will curdle'.[35]

While most menstrual lore proscribed or prohibited some actions, in a few cases there were specific activities prescribed at menarche. In the Philippines, for example, there was a tradition from 'olden days, you have to go on four or five steps, and then you jump. This is signifying something. Maybe they're regulating flow, I don't know, but there's something there so I just followed because my maid told me to do it. I'm panicking you know, I saw blood in my undies. Then my mother came at night time and was told about it and inquired "Have you done it?"'[36] Erlinda recalled her mother telling her 'to jump from the stairs, one-two-three, and I jumped

---

29   Virisila, 11, Fiji 1964.
30   Sue, 13, Singapore 1967.
31   Qing, 12, Hong Kong 1962.
32   Nirmala, 13, Indonesia 1964.
33   Ria, 13, Philippines 1955.
34   Violetta, 14, Philippines 1938.
35   Corazon, 12, Philippines 1956.
36   Ria, 13, Philippines 1955.

because she said it will take three days for your menstruation to flow'.[37] Violetta told me 'they let us slip from the third step of the stairs so the menstruation will be only three days but I did not do that because my mum did not let me'.[38] Corazon, on holiday with her cousins and the centre of their attention, remembered her auntie appearing and asking "'what's going on here?" "Oh", they said, "Corazon's got her period now." "Oh, come, come", she said, "you have to jump [laughing] ... you have to jump from the stairs". We only have a few steps and anyway she said "doesn't matter. You just have to jump from the top down". I don't know how many times, but they just asked me to jump'.[39] Gloria was also directed by her auntie, 'and she tell me to jump. Three times, so the period would not last too long'.[40]

Listening to the menstrual lore of women from such a diversity of cultures provided clear evidence of common themes which fall into in three distinct forms. First, the harmful effect *of* the menstrual body to plant life and certain food preservation processing. Second, the harmful effect of certain substances *to* the menstrual body, internally by ingestion or externally by contact with water. The third theme involved practices at menarche intended to control the menstrual body. I will examine these three forms at greater depth, beginning with Rosalia's statement, which infers a mythical quality with deeper layers to it: 'not all women, but lot of women, have a very strong period and if they touch a plant or a tree it would have died'.[41] Rosalia introduces the binary concept of life and death as women, the givers of life, become the destroyers. She articulates the thought that menstrual power is not universal among women but belongs only to those with a strong period, women perhaps overtaken by a force whose strength is symbolised by pain and flow, breaching the body's boundary to emanate as a separate entity of destruction.

The idea of this destructive power, emerging in a heightened form at menarche and recurring with all subsequent menstrual bleeds, entered Western thought through the writings of Roman naturalist and philosopher Gaius Plinius Secundus, known as Pliny the Elder, who was born in Como in 23 CE. Pliny's *Natural History* combines a written account of the natural world with integrated essays on human achievements and organisation

---

37   Erlinda, 12, Philippines 1964.
38   Violetta, 14, Philippines 1938.
39   Corazon, 12, Philippines 1956.
40   Gloria, 13, Philippines 1959.
41   Rosalia, 13, Italy 1950.

drawn from 100 other works.[42] He emphasises the dangers of 'the power of a menstruous woman', particularly one 'menstruating naturally for the first time', cautioning that 'young vines are irremediably harmed by [her] touch, and rue and ivy, plants of the highest medicinal power, die at once'. Even metal was affected: 'the edge of razors [are] blunted, brass contracts copper rust and a foul smell'.[43] Pliny remained influential in writings about menstrual lore and customs, referenced for example in a 1915 paper by the physician Raymond Crawfurd, on the superstitions of menstruation. Crawfurd cites Pliny's 'seeds which are touched by her become sterile, grafts wither away, garden plants are parched up, and the fruit will fall from the tree beneath which she sits'. In this passage, arguing the threat to fertility by the menstruous woman, Crawfurd perceives the key to women's destructive menstrual force – her power over male virility in the unending struggle over survival of the fittest.[44] Power exists, too, in the context in which Pliny compiled his text, according to Classical historian Lesley Dean-Jones, who claims Pliny's anxiety over the menstruating woman reflects his concern over women's increasing power and autonomy in his own society.[45]

The destructive power of menstruation continued to disturb the men who documented it and centuries later the durability of menstrual lore is seen in the work of British anthropologist-folklorist, Sir James Frazer (1890) who argues that:

> in various parts of Europe, it is still believed that if a woman in her courses enters a brewery the beer will turn sour; if she touches beer, wine, vinegar or milk, it will go bad; if she makes jam it will not keep; if she touches buds, they will wither; if she climbs a cherry tree, it will die.[46]

And in an anonymously written article printed in the prestigious British medical journal *The Lancet*, in 1910, the author points out how menstruating women have historically been regarded in 'a hostile light':

---

42 H. Rackham, 'Introduction', Pliny, *Natural History in Ten Volumes*, vol. 1, trans. H. Rackham, William Heinemann Limited, London 1967, pp. vii–ix.

43 Pliny, *Natural History*, vol. VIII, trans. W. H. S Jones, William Heinemann Limited, London, 1963, p. 57.

44 Pliny, *Natural History*, vol. VII cited in Raymond Crawford, 'Notes on the superstitions of menstruation read before the historical section of the Royal Society of Medicine on Dec. 15th, 1915', *The Lancet*, vol. 186, issue 4816, 18 December 1915, pp. 1332, 1344.

45 Lesley Dean-Jones, *Women's Bodies in Classical Greek Science*, Oxford University Press (1994), Oxford, 2001, pp. 248–249.

46 Sir James Frazer, *The Golden Bough: a Study in Magic and Religion* (1890), abridged edition, vol. II (1922), Macmillan and Company Limited, London, 1957, p. 794.

old-fashioned Wessex and Worcestershire countrywomen, for instance, believed, and perhaps still believe, that when in this condition, they ought not handle raw meat for fear of spoiling it. German peasants, in the same way, believe, according to Ploss (*Das Weib*, 1884), that a menstruous woman entering a cellar turns the wine of the Fatherland to a sourness, and that if she cross a field she spoils the growth of young vegetation.[47]

The beliefs persisted. In 1940 the anthropologist M.F. Ashley-Montagu observed how the great French perfumeries prohibited women working during their periods, and in the famed mushroom-producing areas menstruating women were prohibited from picking. Nor could they work with silkworms in the south of France. Wineries, both in France and in the Rhine area of Germany, forbade menstruating women to be near or to touch any container in which fermentation of was taking place.[48] Even today among Italians living in Toronto menstruating women are considered unsuitable for winemaking or tomato-canning activities; oral historian Luisa del Giudice points out the imitative colour connection with menstrual blood.[49] Closer to home, a science teacher at a private co-educational college in Melbourne, with pupils from diverse ethnic backgrounds, comments on the conviction held by many of her female pupils that:

> they can't pick a lemon from a lemon tree when they have their period. It would poison the tree. Their mother doesn't pick lemon from the lemon tree but would actually wait for the husband or son to come home to do that. Some suggested that you can't water the garden, can't take pickles from the pickle jar, otherwise you spoil the rest ... One of my students even told me 'I don't know if you know Miss but you are not allowed to shower for five days because it stops your period'.[50]

Further examples of belief in the power of menstrual touch are found in Vanuatu, previously the New Hebrides, as Levani from Fiji recalled. Ni-Vanuatu women who were menstruating did not go into the area where young plants were growing, according to feminist literary scholars Janice

---

47   Unknown author, 'The folklore of menstruation', *The Lancet*, vol. 175, issue 4507, 15 January 1910, p. 184.
48   M. F. Ashley-Montagu, 'Physiology and the origin of the menstrual prohibitions', *The Quarterly Review of Biology*, vol. 15, no. 2, 1940, p. 212.
49   Del Giudice, Louisa, 'Wine makes good blood: wine culture among Toronto Italians', http://luisadg.org/wp/wp-content/uploads/2009/11/LGG-Cantina.PDF, p. 18.
50   Sanjakdar (2009), p. 267.

Delaney, Mary Jane Lupton and Emily Toth.[51] Furthermore, Filipino folklore relates that 'if a woman is having her monthly sickness, she should not visit or step on any garden because the plants will turn yellow and it will be destroyed in some way or another'.[52] Similarly, the anthropologist Robert Levy discovered that in the Society Islands of Tahiti, women stayed away from the garden areas while menstruating because of the belief that plants they touched would become diseased, fruit would be ruined and flowers would wilt.[53] More recently, the anthropologist Denise Lawrence, while observing gender relations within the social structure of a small rural town in southern Portugal, found the belief that the contact or even presence of a menstruating woman would cause plants to wilt. Lawrence's work focuses on the effect of the menstruating woman on the socio-economic life of the small town, where gender equality exists in domestic relations and family savings and wealth are invested in pigs. The big event of the year is the annual household slaughter, providing cured meat for family use and for social obligations. The main concern is spoilage by a menstruating woman, whose mere look would cause loss of the source of family protein, money and status. More interesting is the agency women employ within the framework of this belief, which Lawrence argues allows them to maintain a central role in their society. Women are responsible for recruiting additional labour, both male and female, for the annual pig killing and curing activities, and also have control over who enters her property at the time.[54]

Lawrence's research provides evidence that aspects of menstrual lore can still have practical relevance. These tales of the destructive menstrual touch which, like other myths, are usually considered untrue and arise from some past event that resonates with human experience, allow inaccurate claims

---

51 Janice Delaney, Mary Jane Lupton and Emily Toth, *The Curse: a Cultural History of Menstruation* (1976), Revised edition University of Illinois Press, Urbana 1988, p. 11.

52 Francisco Demetrio y Radaza, S. J. (comp. and ed.), *Dictionary of Philippine Folk Beliefs and Customs, Book III*, Xavier University, Cagayan de Oro City 1970, entry 1759, p. 609.

53 Robert L. Levy, *Tahitians: Mind and Experience in the Society Islands*, University of Chicago Press, Chicago 1973, p. 146.

54 Denise Lawrence, 'Menstrual politics: women and pigs in rural Portugal', in *Blood Magic: the Anthropology of Menstruation*, Thomas Buckley and Alma Gottlieb (eds), University of California Press, Berkeley, 1988, pp. 120, 122–123, 125, 128. 'Menstruating women should never salt pigs or enter a dairy or the butter will not churn/the cream will not rise/the cheese will not set' is part of the collection in Mary Chamberlain's *Old Wives' Tales: Their History, Remedies and Spells*, Virago Press Limited, London, 1981, p. 231. Chamberlain gathered the collection of tales from herbal and domestic medical books and folklore and indicates these particular tales have been transmitted orally.

to take on a life of their own in people's minds. The historian Paul Cohen argues that over time, such beliefs can increasingly be accepted as factual, and Lawrence illustrated this by showing how the Portuguese community's belief in the destructive menstrual touch influenced social thought and action, being expressed in certain attitudes and values to serve a particular present and women's role in it.[55] It is the semblance of truth existing in the distorted past event that historians Rebecca Collins and Bain Attwood insist must exist for a myth to form successfully.[56] However, ethno-historian Jan Vansina argues that adaptation or distortion to fit a purpose makes myth an unreliable source, despite the fact that it remains central to the world-view of any culture.[57] Most important, in the context of menstrual touch, is the accuracy of Cohen's observation that myth assumes its most bizarre characteristics when historical evidence is absent.[58]

Without historical evidence the mythical quality of menstrual lore presents problems for interpretation. How are we to 'read' the stories of threat to lemon and mango trees and to other plant life, and what do we make of the menstrual power to ruin a year's supply of vital sauce? At the 13th Katherine Briggs Memorial Lecture, in 1994, anthropologist Mary Douglas presented a paper discussing the interpretation of stories and myths, arguing that when social context is missing, meaning is attributed afresh by each new reader or listener who will, by habit, seek to interpret the original intention. Citing a French version of the familiar tale of Red Riding Hood as a vehicle for interpretation Douglas shows how understanding comes through cultural knowledge. More generally, Douglas surmises that folktales mirror life as it was, as a commentary on a current happening, and that the world of women was in reality a world of 'blood, sex and rivalry' in which beliefs about female physiology were transmitted from generation to generation. In myth and folktale the bodies of women are constructed as a contradiction to those of men. In opposition to men's isolation from the cycles of nature, women have monthly menstrual cycles equating to Nature's year, swinging them between emotion and rationality, mirroring Nature's

---

55   Paul A. Cohen, *History in Three Keys: the Boxers as Event, Experience, and Myth*, Columbia University Press, New York 1997, pp. 211–215.

56   Rebecca Collins, 'Concealing the poverty of traditional historiography: myth as mystification in historical discourse', *Rethinking History* vol. 7, no. 3, 2003, p. 343 and Bain Attwood, *Possession: Batman's Treaty and the Matter of History*, Miegunyah Press, Carlton 2009, p. 121.

57   Jan Vansina, *Oral Tradition: a Study in Historical Methodology* (1965), trans. H.M. Wright, Routledge and Keegan Paul, London, 1969, pp. 156–157.

58   Cohen (1997), p. 214.

seasons of fermentation, budding, laying and proliferating. Their work is focused on the body in birthing, feeding, bathing and caring, and Douglas suggests that it was women's recognition of connection between their own bodies and the natural world that caused them to impose restrictions on themselves. By avoiding touching fermenting wine, or pork curing in brine, they prevented any destructive bodily contagion caused by their like-state.[59]

Douglas argues that every time we read myth or folklore we try to locate the original meaning, and Cohen argues for the association between myth and human experience. I have found both in my many readings about menstrual lore and the widely shared belief in the dangers of menstrual touch. Looking for a missing link to help explain the centuries-old belief, I considered both the context and the conditions of women's labour. The ordinary tasks of a woman's daily life may not have held any significance in transmission of menstrual lore, nor to the men who later wrote the myths, but there is relevance. For instance, Lawrence has given the example that culturally and historically women did not slaughter animals. Their job was the preparation of meat for keeping through the salting and curing processes. In Italy they helped harvest, prepare and cook the tomatoes. In other countries their labour followed similar patterns. The work was arduous, requiring physical exertion over fires for long hours, day after day, during late summer and autumn. Often these women worked in conditions which made them sweat profusely. Hence they produced the physical circumstances that subsequent scientific research has theorised is necessary for the secretion of menstrual toxin. (This research is discussed later in the chapter.) It can also be argued women's menarche and menstruation produced the political circumstances necessary for collective action by providing an interlude from their labour, one justified and maintained through myth. Moreover, the significance of myth in inter-group relations includes the propaganda value for men of the group, who could claim power through association, in relating the myth. So the story of menarcheal and menstrual power, and its effect on plants and meat processing, remains alive in some cultures until change, through education and technology, removes the need for it, committing it to the memories of old women and the perpetuity of writing.

The second form of menstrual lore is cautionary, warning of the harmful effect of certain substances *to* the menstrual body, internally through ingestion of certain foods and externally by contact with water. Once again,

---

59   Mary Douglas, 'Red Riding Hood: an interpretation from anthropology', *Folklore*, vol. 106, 1995, pp. 1, 4–5.

scientific research has provided certain validation for this age-old belief. Although many young girls, such as the Singapore-born Chinese Sue, were educated in a modern system, women's menstrual lore remained influential. Sue clearly recalled her mother's succinct 'no eating of stuff like pineapple'. Similarly in Sri Lanka, foods including pineapple, pawpaw and mango were avoided due to the belief that they cause extreme blood loss and cramping pain, with Malays and Chinese in Malaysia believing pineapple to have abortifacient properties.[60] In Haiti, Yolette Garaud, who experienced her menarche at 10 years of age, learned that:

> A girl past eight years old was not supposed to eat certain fruit, like pineapple. Anything that was sour was a no-no. When I asked my grandmother why, she told me it was because at that age a girl's body is changing and those fruits interfere with certain chemicals, and that death could be the result of such interference. Not knowing better, I just swallowed the story. Years after, I discovered it was just one of the thousands of myths surrounding menstruation.[61]

In her study of food beliefs and critical life events in peninsular Malaysia, medical anthropologist Lenore Manderson found pineapple, considered to be sharp and cold, was the most cited food cause of heavy menstrual flow and pain.[62] Once again, scientific study has endorsed that which women in pineapple-growing areas have long known. The stem and fruit of the pineapple plant contains the substance bromelain, which has been tested as an anti-inflammatory agent for use in various medical conditions. On of the side-effects listed is menstrual problems: 'bromelain may cause abnormal uterine bleeding or heavy/prolonged menstruation'.[63] Its supplementary use for dysmenorrhoea, or painful periods, is noted in a UK hospital information sheet:

> Bromelain: an enzyme found in pineapples, which has exceptional anti-inflammatory and blood thinning properties. Also relaxes smooth muscle (the uterus is made of smooth muscle) and increases the

---

60 Chandrani Weerasinghe, Srikanthi Karaliedde, T. W. Wikramanayake, 'Food beliefs and practices among Sri Lankans: temporary food avoidances by women', *Journal of the National Science Council of Sri Lanka*, vol. 10, no. 1, 1982, p. 61, 63–64.

61 Yolette Garaud, 'A student's journal: on menstruation', *Women's Studies Newsletter*, vol. 6, no. 3, 1978, p. 23.

62 Lenore Manderson, 'Traditional food beliefs and critical life events in Peninsular Malaysia', *Social Science Information* vol. 20, no. 6, 1981, pp. 964–965.

63 'Drugs and supplements: Bromelain', http:// www.nlm.nih.gov/medlineplus/print/ druginfo/natural/patient-bromelain.html

production of 'good' prostaglandins while reducing the production of 'bad' ones.[64]

It might be asked which comes first, menstrual pain that modern day Western institutions treat with bromelain from pineapple, or the heavy menstrual flow that bromelain causes? Evidence suggests wisdom in the menstrual lore of avoidance.

Sue had been instructed on the effect certain foods had on menstrual blood coagulation and on traditional Chinese 'heating-cooling' foods, which she did not elaborate on. Qing recalled advice from her sister about the effect of cold drinks on menstrual pain. According to sociologist Cordia Chu, who researched the menstrual beliefs of 97 Chinese women with diverse geographic and economic backgrounds from Hong Kong and the People's Republic of China, there is a general conformity to the underlying principles of *yin-yang* relating to concepts of cold-hot during menstruation, but some regional variation in defining which foods are cold in nature, and no reference made to the exotic pineapple. Chu argues that at menarche and during menstruation female bodies are significantly under the influence of the cold principle, *yin*, causing systemic imbalance, so any substances which exacerbate imbalance should be avoided. Women are advised against temperature-cold yin foods because they are thought to impair blood flow, with resultant pain. Conversely, foods cold in nature are thought to cause excessively heavy blood flow and are to be avoided. Maintaining the yin-yang harmony is endorsed by the People's Republic of China in public health information texts advising women against eating sour, salty, or cold foods while menstruating, advice still considered important by Chinese trained in Western medicine.[65]

In north-east Thailand, girls at menarche hear about food avoidance and how menstrual blood, considered a 'hot' substance, can emanate a heat that harms plants classified as 'cool' (such as mint). Thai menstrual lore includes anecdotes about the ingestion of cold-temperature foods, which obstruct menstrual flow, forcing it to the head and bringing about insanity.[66] They

---

64 'Dysmenorrhoea', *Patient Information*, Basildon and Thurrock University Hospitals, http://www.basildonandthurrock.nhs.uk

65 Cordia Ming-Yeuk Chu, 'Menstrual beliefs and practices of Chinese Women', *Journal of the Folklore Institute*, vol. 17, no. 1, 1980, pp. 41–44. See also Charlotte Furth and Ch'en Shu-Yeuh, 'Chinese medicine and the anthropology of menstruation in contemporary Taiwan', *Medical Anthropology Quarterly*, vol. 6, no. 1, 1992, p. 36.

66 Andrea Whittaker, *Intimate Knowledge: Women and their Health in North-east Thailand*, Allen and Unwin, St Leonards 2000, pp. 72–74.

share the belief in humoral physiology with Malays, and have similar hot-cold food classification and avoidances at menarche and during menstruation.[67] Menstrual lore related by Filipino women was notably alike in the belief that food high in acid prevented good blood flow. Repeatedly, they related that at menarche girls were told not to eat green mangoes and to avoid anything containing vinegar.

The link between menstrual flow and the ingestion of certain foods was widely believed. In Chile menarcheal girls were told to avoid lemon, as we have seen. Spanish-speaking Lola's explanation of cause and effect, based on the cultural practice of adding lemon juice to the blood of a freshly slaughtered lamb for keeping purposes, is based on the scientific principles of objectivity and reproducibility but appear physiologically skewed in the action of ingested lemon juice on the menstrual process. Nevertheless the belief was widespread, with Maria in Italy relating that she too had been told to avoid lemon because of its effects on her menstrual blood flow. Among Mayan women in Chichimila, Mexico, the anthropologist Yewoubdar Beyene found the same avoidance of lemons for the same reason: the congealing effect on menstrual blood.[68] The cautionary purpose of this form of menstrual lore was to ensure menstrual health as an indicator of good general health, hence reproductive health, among women of many cultures as we have seen above.

Equally of concern was the effect of water on the body of the menarcheal girl or the menstruating woman. A medical guide for women published in Canada in 1901 illustrates this concern:

> Great care should be used to guard against any influences that may tend to derange the menses. Sudden suppression is always dangerous. Cold baths, foot baths, wetting the feet by the wearing of thin shoes, are very injurious during this period. A young woman anxious to attend a party or ball during this period sometimes takes a hip bath to arrest the discharge, but what a train of horrors follows such an insane act, and still there are many foolish enough to do this. [69]

The 'train of horrors' risked by socially active girl, was a 'cold of the uterus' that might progress to chronic uterine inflammation, of major concern in

67   Manderson (1981), pp. 949–950.
68   Yewoubdar Beyene, *From Menarche to Menopause: Reproductive Lives of Peasant Women in Two Cultures*, State University of New York Press, Albany, 1989, pp. 105–106.
69   Mary R. Melendy, *Perfect Womanhood for Maidens – Wives – Mothers*, World Publishing Company, Guelph, Ontario, 1901, pp. 93, 182.

Western societies at the time. Menarcheal girls worldwide to be cautioned about the effects of water on the menstrual body, but with diverse reasons based on different vulnerabilities. Maryam in Lebanon believed that water on her head endangered her health because during menstruation her blood vessels were open, making her vulnerable to infection, and in Taiwan today the same concept of vulnerability is present in women's belief that bathing makes the menstrual body vulnerable to germs.[70] In the Philippines, Ria was told just to sponge and clean herself but never to get cold water in her vagina. Marjorie in England also associated water on the menstrual body with unwellness, recalling how menstruating girls were excused from swimming classes at school. Cold water was associated with menstrual pain according to Maria in Italy and Virsilia in Fiji, and with the effect on menstrual flow by Ramona and Lola in Chile.

In Alexandria, Nadia was told that washing her body would cause heavy bleeding, and in Ukraine Olena's grandmother told her that hot baths would have the same effect. In the Philippines attitudes to water varied. The belief that wetting the head caused craziness, as Corazon related, is also part of English folklore, which attributes 'brain fever' to hair washing.[71] Aleli remembered being told that cold water on the menstrual body would predispose her to later rheumatism. Showering was prohibited for seven days.[72] Ria and Erlinda recalled a three-day prohibition on showering, and a collection of Filipino folk-medicine proscriptions recommends the menarcheal girl or menstruating woman 'should not take a bath for if she does the blood would stop flowing.[73] The belief that bathing causes menstrual pain remains present in parts of the Philippines.[74] In every directive of this menstrual lore is the same purpose as that of food avoidance: menstrual health signified by flow as an indicator of women's reproductive health. When that becomes controlled by other means, including socio-cultural shifts and education, the significance of this menstrual lore may be lost.

---

70 Furth and Shu-Yueh (1992), p. 37.
71 Chamberlain (1981), p. 231. See also Daryl Costos, Ruthie Ackerman and Lisa Paradis, 'Recollections of menarche: communication between mothers and daughters regarding menstruation', *Sex Roles*, vol. 46, nos 1–2, 2002, p. 54.
72 I have encountered this among Chinese women immediately post-partum.
73 Francisco Demetrio y Radaza, S.J., (comp. and ed.), *Dictionary of Philippine Folk Beliefs and Customs, Book II,*(1970), Xavier University, Cagayan de Oro City 1970, entry 1390, p. 443.
74 World Health Organisation Western Pacific Region, 'Sexual and reproductive health of adolescents and youths in the Philippines: a review of literature and projects 1995–2003', Office of Publications, World Health Organisation, Geneva, 2005, p. 64.

The third form of menstrual lore, described at the beginning of the chapter, told of certain activities performed at menarche in the Philippines that were intended to control the duration of future menstrual periods. This prescribed activity has a firm place in Filipino folk-medicine and is reported by health professionals, working among adolescent girls in Mindanao, as one of the intergeneration transmissions of menstrual lore carried out 'for the sake of tradition'.

On the day of a girl's first menstruation, she must jump over three steps of the stairs. This will limit her menstruation to three days afterwards.[75]

This and the other aspects of menstrual lore recalled by my interviewees has been part of women's knowledge for over 2,000 years. It is gender specific, usually transmitted by older family members – grandmothers, mothers, aunts or sisters – at the occasion of menarche and takes three identifiable forms, each relating to power. In the first instance, the overt purpose is the transmission of belief that harmful and destructive power begins emanating from the menstrual body at menarche, necessitating prohibition of certain physical actions for the protection of specified matter. The covert purpose of this form of lore is the transmission of agency that women have from the effects of their power, allowing them an intermission from their labour, particularly for women in non-industrialised areas. The second form of menstrual lore transmits the belief that the menstrual body is vulnerable to the harmful power of certain matter entering the body internally, through ingestion, or externally through contact. The third form combines the transmission of belief with prescribed, and supervised, physical action intended to generate power over the menarcheal body through control of blood flow. While scientific research into aspects of the first two forms has produced data indicating that certain menstrual lore may be based on observable fact, there is nothing for the third form which remains somewhat anomalous in its cultural practice and containment. However, it must be remembered that for all but one interviewee English was a second language, and for many fluency was lacking, so that menstrual lore told in regional dialects may 'read' differently. Nonetheless, there is a notable uniformity of belief among the individual Filipino participants who reiterated the event, cultural practice and intended effect.

---

75 WHO Western Pacific Region, 'Sexual and reproductive health of adolescents and youths in the Philippines: a review of literature and projects 1995–2003' (2005), p. 64.

Although there are noteworthy similarities and a broad cross-cultural global distribution in the menstrual lore related, it is not nationally widespread in the countries represented and some Italian interviewees, for example, were either unfamiliar with, or disbelieving of, stories told by other Italian women in the group. Characteristic of the genres of myth and folklore, the shared similarities include lack of context, particularly chronological, making historical interpretation and explanation of meaning in the conventional sense almost impossible. Although menstrual lore was, and remains in some cultures, 'owned' by women in the oral tradition, English language and literature scholar Christine Neufeld argues that the advent of literacy enabled men, with the authority of education, to document the lore as 'old wives' tales' in the subversive context of gender politics, evident in assertions made by the authors about women, who were their sources of information.[76] Overall, the purpose of menstrual lore, which goes back to ancient times in every culture, is to protect women's reproductive health. Today, menstrual lore has almost disappeared in the industrialised world except among recently arrived immigrant communities, where women enforce certain cultural beliefs perceived to benefit young girls, or where transmission through other media is presented as part of a bigger picture of menarche and menstruation.

As part of the bigger picture, the place of scientific investigation into the phenomenon of the destructive power of the menarcheal or menstruating woman deserves acknowledgement. In 1920 the paediatrician Bela Schick, whose name would later become known through the Schick test for susceptibility to diphtheria, received a bunch of fresh roses that his attendant was reluctant to handle. Insisting that they be put in a vase of water, she complied. The roses wilted shortly afterwards and, in discussing their condition, Schick learned the woman was menstruating and her reluctance to handle the flowers was because she anticipated the effect from previous occurrences. Curious, Schick followed up historical sources on the subject, including Pliny, and, challenged by general opinion that the destructive power of menstruation was nothing more than superstition, decided to test the matter. He demonstrated that during the first two days of menstruation an unidentified toxic substance circulated in the blood and was excreted through the skin, including the hands. Its effect on flowers was found to be prevented by the use of sterile gloves. In another test, using a minimal

---

76   Christine Neufeld, 'Speakerly women and scribal men', *Oral Tradition*, vol. 14, no. 2, 1999, pp. 420–421, 426.

amount of circulating blood, Schick found the growth of yeast was inhibited. When not menstruating, women's blood produced no change.[77] However, in his 1940 paper Ashley-Montagu refers to 'certain women' having the destructive menstrual power, which links with Rosalia's conviction that it was not homogeneous.[78]

Other scientific investigations followed. In 1923 pharmacologists David I. Macht and Dorothy S. Lubin, using living plants in their research into toxicology, tested bodily secretions from healthy menstruating women.[79] In all cases their results indicated that immediately pre-menstrual, and during the first two days of a period, levels of toxicity were evident in menstrual saliva, in skin secretion from the hands, which showed variations in levels of toxicity between individuals, and in axillary sweat.[80] Blood products tested included serum, showing significant variation in toxicity between individuals with the highest levels obtained from young girls at and just post-menarche; red blood cells; and whole blood, which proved the most toxic of all. Additionally, whole dry blood and dry menstrual blood were tested and shown to retain their toxic properties,[81] something of significance in Chinese belief, where it was believed to be dangerous to walk on the streets because of the possible presence of dry menstrual blood.[82] A decade later, in 1934, medical researchers William Freeman and Joseph Looney modified the methods used by Macht and Lubin, to test the blood of healthy women for further evidence of menstrual toxin. The blood was taken within three days from the start of a period, usually

---

77 Horace L. Hodes, 'Introduction to the presentation of the John Howland medal and award of the American Pediatric Society to Dr Bela Schick', *AMA American Journal of Diseases of Children*, vol. 89. no. 2, 1955, pp. 248–249. See also Rita M. Montgomery, 'A cross-cultural study of menstruation, menstrual taboos, and related social variables', *Ethos*, vol. 2, no. 2, 1974, p. 144; Thomas Buckley and Alma Gottlieb, 'A critical appraisal of theories of menstrual symbolism', in Thomas Buckley and Alma Gottlied (eds) *Blood Magic: the Anthropology of Menstruation*, University of California Press, Berkeley 1988, p. 20; and Delaney et al (1988), p. 12.

78 Ashley-Montagu (1940), p. 214.

79 David L. Macht and Dorothy S. Lubin, 'A phyto-pharmacological study of menstrual toxin', *Journal of Pharmacology and Experimental Therapeutics*, vol. 22, no. 5, 1923, p. 414.

80 Macht and Lubin (1923), pp. 418–419, 427–430.

81 Macht and Lubin (1923), pp. 421–426. Macht and Lubin also found evidence of toxicity in breast milk from menstruating women who were understandably difficult to find. See p. 430–431. It has long been observed by women, myself included, that babies may suffer gastrointestinal discomfort for a day or so. This has been confirmed by V. R. Pickles. See Vernon R. Pickles, 'Prostaglandins and dysmenorrhoea: historical survey', *Acta Obstetricia et Gynecologia Scandanavia*, vol. 58, no. S87, 1979, p. 7.

82 Buckley and Gottlieb (1988), in Buckley and Gottlieb (eds), pp. 34–35.

the first day, and again mid-cycle. Their findings showed no increased toxicity at menstruation.[83]

Research continuing through the 1930s convinced Ashley-Montagu that 20th-century science had seemingly explained the long-held idea that menstruating women were imbued with a power destructive to plant life and other matter.[84] It appears that the war years may have reduced both opportunity and interest in further research but in the 1970s references to menstrual toxin reappeared in the British medical journal *Lancet*, with Dr Helen Reid commented on 'the brass-ring sign', a black stain under the gold rings worn by women, attributed to skin secretion immediately before menstruation or during the first two days of a period.[85] Dr Reid's observation, with its shades of Pliny, caused Dr Geoffrey Davis to ask 'what is this stuff?' drawing attention to the fact that although the pharmacological basis for menstrual toxin had been provided by Schick, Macht and Lubin, identity of the actual agent remained unknown.[86] The physiologist Vernon Pickles argued that although toxic to certain plants, menstrual toxin was less harmful to animal tissue. Pickles speculated on the possibility that it may belong to the group of prostaglandins, linking it to premenstrual depression, and called for further investigation.[87] He later interested botanists in the subject, arguing the need for a better plant-test system to enable isolation of menstrual toxin, now referred to as menotoxin. With J. A. Bryant and D. G. Heathcote, Pickles tested menstrual fluid from students not taking oral contraceptives and found evidence of accelerated deterioration of Kalanchöe flowers. They were unable to isolate menotoxin from the many prostaglandins, and conjectured that it may not be a single substance, or emanate only from the menstruating uterus, but might instead be a substance or substances linked with menstrual mood instability.[88] From then on, little

---

83   William Freeman and Joseph M. Looney with the technical assistance of Rose R. Small, 'Studies on the phytotoxic index: II. menstrual toxin ("Menotoxin") from the Worcester State Hospital and the Memorial Foundation for Neuro-Endocrine Research Worcester, Massachusetts', *Journal of Pharmacological and Experimental Therapeutics*, vol. 52, no. 2, 1934, pp. 179–183.

84   Ashley-Montagu (1940), p. 217.

85   Helen Evans Reid, 'The brass-ring sign', *Lancet*, vol. 303, issue 7864, 18 May 1974, p. 988.

86   Geoffrey Davis, '"Menstrual toxin" and human fertility', *Lancet*, vol. 303, issue 7867, 8 June 1974, p. 1192.

87   V. R. Pickles, '"Menstrual toxin" again', *Lancet*, vol. 303, issue 7869, 22 June 1974, pp. 1292–1293.

88   J. A. Bryant, D.G. Heathcote, V. R. Pickles, 'The search for "menotoxin"', *The Lancet*, vol. 309, issue 18014, 2 April 1977, p. 753. See also Buckley and Gottlieb (1988), in Buckley and Gottlieb (eds), pp. 19–20 and their criticism of Schick et al's theory, which is based on cultural practice unrelated to the argument constructed.

was heard about menotoxin, although the gynaecologist Nelson Soucasaux maintains there is some truth in the old stories of the destructive power of the menarcheal or menstruating woman. He points out that prostaglandins are present in the endometrium, the uterine lining which breaks down as menstrual blood, and these are responsible for menstrual contractions. As a result, Soucasaux argues a connection between menotoxins, which remain an unidentified substance or substances, and prostaglandins, stressing that the body which produces many toxic substances must constantly excrete them to enable maintenance of normal blood chemistry levels.[89]

Conclusion

In view of the current understanding of physiology, and the highly sophisticated research equipment that makes possible an exploration of connection between the menstruating body and traditional menstrual lore, it almost seems a pity that the whole phenomenon of menstrual lore is disappearing. It could be argued, though, to have outlived its purpose in today's world. The purpose being control, practised in two ways: control of knowledge relating to the menstruating body by older women, and transmitted to a girl at menarche; and control by the girl, according to instructions received, over certain activities during menstruation, and in one example given by interviewees, activities by a girl to control duration of menstruation. The relationship between the transmission and reception of the lore, constructed in the transformative state of menarche, communicated to the girl that women's menstruating bodies were both powerful, and vulnerable to malevolent power, particularly at menarche.

The survival of women's lore was evident in the interview data and indicated the wide cultural spectrum of its history as well as the similarities in form and content, told as brief anecdotes of a prohibitive nature, and including some Mediterranean lore recognisable from the writings of Pliny in 32 C.E. indicating an ancient existence.

Interview data showed a wide variation in women's understanding of the rationale behind the prohibitions and avoidances they described. No one mentioned 'menotoxin' although it was perhaps alluded to by several women in their references to 'strong periods' of potentially toxic affect. Chemical intervention has meant that menstrual problems are in general less a part of menstrual life for women than they were in the past. Indeed,

---

89   Nelson Soucasaux, 'Menstrual toxin: an old name for a real thing?'
      http://www.mum.org/menotox2.htm 2001.

the growing tendency toward chemically controlled menstruation may well prevent further investigation into a biological explanation for the rationale behind menstrual lore and belief in the destructive power of menarche and menstruation. Yet while myths are transmitted orally, visually, or in writing, human curiosity about the event or experience that attributes young girls and women with a supernatural power will almost certainly remain, so, too, will menstrual lore be kept alive by folklorists in oral presentation and writing. Although there may be no further scientific study into the phenomena of the menstrual touch, or investigations into the effect of certain foods eaten during menarche and menstruation, the subject will maintain historic relevance because of its glimpse across the centuries into human thought, and the ways in which diverse cultures made almost identical meanings about the process that begins at menarche.

Chapter 6

CONCEALING THE FACT

Sometimes in the street I saw girls having the stain on their dress.
They can't avoid it.[1]

Among the culturally diverse interviewees, a shared concern was that of successfully concealing menstruation, particularly at menarche, and many reflected on the difficulties this caused. Although well removed from the days of adapting mosses or fibres to act as menstrual absorbents, the burden of making and caring for menstrual paraphernalia from a fairly young age anticipated the harsher lives of adult women in many cultures. One repeated feature of menarche was the help and advice women gave to each other about managing menstrual life. In many cases older women were the only educators and their attitudes toward menstruation, both positive and negative, were transmitted with their guidance. While recalling the memories, my informants became young girls once again, experiencing menarche many years ago in their countries of birth. Most are now grandmothers, living in a different culture, recreating the world of their youth and the physical practices and cultural values that surrounded an experience through which many of them come to be seen as young women.

The interview data provided by these women makes clear the extent to which menarche and menstruation belonged to a female realm, although as we have seen in earlier chapters, these specifically female aspects of culture and ritual occurred in a framework in which men exercised the wider social and religious control over menarcheal and menstrual bleeding. For the majority of women the concealment of bleeding, beginning at menarche, followed customary methods that involved some curtailment of activity external to the home. There was no thought of protest against this and no suggestion that it might change. Modern sanitary hygiene practice in

---

1   Qing, 12 years old at menarche, Hong Kong 1962.

Western countries, however, did reflect changes in the position of women, including young women's access to higher education, greater participation in the public space through employment, and the effects of two world wars. However, there were other significant factors as well, including an increasing medical focus on bodily hygiene and scientific and technological developments that made female hygiene into an industry.

Interview data emphasises the importance of concealing menstrual blood for women from non-industrialised countries, and the effects of this concealment on the women themselves. For instance, Yunuva shared the memories of her 11-year-old self in transit from Egypt to Australia in 1957, her existing migratory stresses enhanced by the onset of menarche in Genoa. Although Yanuva had her mother and older sister to help her through the trauma, she recalled with horror the accoutrements of her changed condition, which her mother provided. She remembers being 'presented with this pad which was made of ... like ... linen sort of fabric with terry-towelling on top, and it had the shape of being a long ... long rectangle with a triangle on either end, and at each side of the triangle there was a loop. And then you had this long piece of ... like a belt made out of fabric and you strap it in and you put it all around'.[2] Yanuva describes the adult-sized menstrual harness, applied to her small body, that was the introduction to life as a menstruating woman for so many young girls, and which became symbolic of menstrual restriction and discomfort. At a similar time in Manila, Corazon discovered that her first high school project was one with a difference, being both practical and beneficial in the way it opened a forum for discussion among her classmates. She recalled that 'when we reach high school the girls start to make their own pads. We were taught. That's the first project we do. You have to make your own pads ... made of cotton, cotton cloth, and boiled. There is a pattern that you sew and then you make a belt'. In answer to a question about commercially made pads Corazon replied, 'no. No we don't. Sometimes we have to cut old cotton shirts and things like that, and that is what we use'.[3] Aleli, who was younger than Corazon at menarche and probably still in primary school, said nothing about pad-making as a high school project, remembering only that 'in 1959 sanitary pads were not really popular yet. We have things like a binder made of muslin cloth, the brown one like they use for the baby ... it's a soft fabric and you have to fold it and fold it and

2   Yanuva, 10, Egypt 1957.
3   Corazon, 12, Philippines 1956.

then clip it to a belt … and then wash it'.[4] The story had been much the same in Sicily for Rosalia, who observed that 'in those days there wasn't anything to buy and Mum used to buy material and make them … I don't know if it was the same here'.[5] No, it was not the same in Australia, but it was in Ukraine, where 'they made their own cloths. They did it themselves from the material because we didn't have such things like here. We washed them'.[6]

In Korea, Jung discovered that 'my mother made already, in case, some pads … gauze … long ones and she folded it and made them. We have to wash them'.[7] Sun, in Seoul, explained 'there were no pads here'.[8] Maryam remembered 'cloths like face washers laundered in boiling water like baby nappies'.[9] In Suva, Levani tried to maintain her privacy at menarche, explaining 'my mother did a lot of sewing so I just went to her box and gathered scraps of material. I was very lucky in that but I had to make sure that I chose the ones she wouldn't miss. I went and had a shower and came back with just a little strip of material and when I got up the blood had gone right through … because we sit on the floor… when I got up my mother saw the blood and she just said to me "look at your sulu", so I did that and then realised the blood was on it so I went … nothing else was said … I went to the bathroom and cleaned myself up and when I came back she had this thing she wears which is like half a nappy, with two holders like loops, and I had no idea what these things were although I'd seen them hanging on the line. She just said "this is what you do" and she showed me how to fold it and then stick it under the pocket thing and then you loop it around, you tie a string around it and I thought "that's interesting" so that day I wore it and felt so uncomfortable that I said to myself I'll never wear it again and I never did'.[10]

Levani had choice because 'in Fiji you just ask for money from friends and sisters, and like I said, I had two older sisters so I just told them I needed money and they gave me … I didn't tell them I was having my period'. As a result, she was able to purchase disposable pads. But not all women could do that, and the interviewees who lacked the opportunity seemed more accepting of being in close contact with their menstrual blood, through

---

4   Aleli, 10, Philippines 1959.
5   Rosalia, 13, Italy 1950.
6   Alla, 14, Ukraine, year unknown, and Kateryna, 15, Ukraine 1952.
7   Jung, 13, South Korea 1959.
8   Sun, 13, South Korea 1962.
9   Maryam, 15, Lebanon 1942.
10   Levani, 16, Fiji 1967.

washing their cloths or pads. Although some interviewees described pads made from specifically chosen fabric, Corazon alluded to the necessity of cutting up old clothes and other interviewees described the ways in which they made use of what was available for absorbing the menstrual flow. Rara, in Jogjakarta, made the point by demonstrating with paper serviettes how she would fold old material to make a menstrual pad from 'cloths, cloths, old cloth. My grandma tells me that sometime, because I not very smart, sometime I put pin in pant and the pin stuck open, in me [much laughter from friends]'. The cloths were thrown away 'because this is old cloth'.[11] This statement was discussed among the group, most of whom agreed that menstrual cloths were washed and reused. Nirmala recalled her menarche in Jogjakarta, over a decade later, when many Indonesian women still made their own pads. 'We grew up in a simple way of life so old cloth like batik just torn off and we make like some sort of parcel with the thick part [demonstrates a roll] just like that. We have another long material to wrap it in. The thick part is where the blood goes through. My mum gave me a belt of material and then the long part you put over and then we put a safety pin in there. When it's all very wet we have to wash them and hang them so we have two or three. Because it's not a wealthy family we can't afford to buy. My friend from a wealthy family would buy some sort of towelling material but even then they still have to wash them and hang them. Nothing got thrown away'.[12]

Poverty determined the level of menstrual hygiene. In Lucknow, Hetal, who was motherless, lived with her extended family, which included several women. She explained that at menarche 'I have the liberty to have a cloth and put on. I have lots to try, that's one advantage we have, and sometime next day I find this cloth, and a new cloth just after that, after some time the squat I use because in market no nappies, no nappies. At that time no cotton'.[13] Nevertheless, Hetal also had some awareness of the strategy used by women who were deprived of even rags to absorb menstrual blood. Saha elaborated, remembering that in Bangalore 'we used to see the ladies sitting on the gunny bags. We're wondering why. They said they're sick. We said when you're sick why would you sit on a gunny bag? It never occurred to me that this was the reason they were sitting for three days, with long blouses just covering themselves ... pads were not rampant in those times. You had

---

11   Rara, 12, Indonesia 1951.
12   Nirmala, 13, Indonesia 1964.
13   Hetal, 14, India c.1952.

to tear old clothes and old sheets and even wash them and re-use them. This is what happens in places where you don't have these pads sold'.[14]

And there were many such places – including Uganda. Cecile explained 'because we didn't have pads we were using cloth from old linen',[15] which introduced the problem of physical discomfort recalled by Ruth. 'I got used to the habit of putting thick tissues because there were no pads like now we have commercial pads but in those days you had to improvise. Maybe tear pieces of cloth and put together and one thing I realised was during period time I got hurt, really, because when you put pad material, and you're walking, you're really rubbing and you get bruised and hurt. You didn't have actual pads to help so when [a period] caught you without any extra cloths to put on you could easily be messed up'. Ruth related a social occasion when she was travelling to a wedding with a group of young people. 'I realised I had started to have this thing… and the whole day I felt so uneasy and we had to travel in this little truck where we have so many young men as well and we didn't have seats … we had to squat the whole way. It was messy and I was holding myself saying "what is going to happen?" I thought everybody thought "what a dirty girl"'.[16]

Being 'messed up' was a shared dread for these women, many speaking of alternative ways to cope with their menstrual flow, including using readily discarded paper. Zosime, in Alexandria, emphasised, 'poor family, you know? No pads. I was working and it was very hard. I use toilet paper'.[17] Elena demonstrated: 'see what happens in making pads from toilet paper'.[18] Melena, in Santiago, recalled 'Mum folded toilet paper and said "you start this and then you get back and you change"'.[19] Lee, in Singapore, described learning about menstruation as she assisted her mother to prepare for her next period. 'My mother's a very quiet sort of lady from a different era, born in the early nineteen something and when I was young, at about nine years old I bought the papers for her and helped her with the folding'. Lee told me that the papers were bought by the pound weight, around 500 grams. She continued: 'the folding was like a fan. It would be quite long and we'll fold it like a fan and then fold it in half, and I remember she had a piece of cloth where she used it around and there were sort of things she could tuck the

14   Saha, 13, India year unknown.
15   Cecile, 16, Uganda 1965.
16   Ruth, 17, Uganda c.1974.
17   Zosime, 11, Egypt 1934.
18   Elena, 14, Greece, year unknown.
19   Melena, 14, Chile, year unknown.

paper in between. The paper was very thin, not as thick as blotting paper because if it's too thick if you fold it'll crack'.[20] Qing made it clear that 'we can go on our normal life as usual as long as we put on the protective gearing. It is traditional, unlike the pad we use today. We use tissue just like the Chinese tissue paper. Before that we have to do preparations, you know, crumple them and then make piles to put in the underpants with plastic to support it. You wash your stained clothing or underpants separately. Not to mix with the family's washing because it was something not polite'.[21] For both women the use of paper appeared traditional as much as economic but for Bao in Saigon it was different. 'We have paper. Very hard but the Vietnamese very poor, you know. Have not got the money to buy the pads, but the toilet paper's very hard, not like here, and we roll, roll to a pad and use a little plastic bit put in the middle, and this is like a pad, you know'.[22]

Throughout this time commercial disposable pads were available but they seemed very large for small bodies. Malaya brought this to mind, remembering that we 'had the Kotex pads. They used to be very bulky things and you had to buy the sanitary belt and my mother taught me how to put it on'.[23] Gloria, in Manila, remembered 'we just had the made ones'.[24] In Santiago, Ramona had very negative memories. 'I never liked my period, especially on a hot day and having to go to school with that in place, because I am so heavy I have to use very, very strong Modess. That part was ... I hate it. I hate it'.[25] Sue, in Singapore, 'remembered there was Kotex, there was Modess, those were the two I knew of'.[26] In Concepcion, Lola recalled the cultural emphasis placed on women's hymenal virginity: 'we didn't have tampons. No'.[27] However, the woman who summarised a wider experience of sanitary protection, and the only one to mention the use of tampons, was Marjorie in England. My mother said "I haven't got any sanitary towels in. You'll have to make do" and gave me this lump of rag with two big safety pins. In those days we used to wear very thick knickers, like flannelette almost, so you were secure. You weren't really going to drip anywhere because it would have been absorbed. That night my mother gave me a sanitary belt. I know it

20   Lee, 13, Singapore 1962.
21   Qing, 12, Hong Kong 1962.
22   Bao, 12, Vietnam 1968.
23   Malaya, 12, Philippines 1956.
24   Gloria, 13. Philippines 1959.
25   Ramona, 15, Chile 1964.
26   Sue, 13, Singapore 1967.
27   Lola, 17, Chile 1967.

was elastic and I think the Dr White's sanitary towels hooked on to a hook. I remember it being very uncomfortable indeed and it all seemed to be a trial to me. Having two older sisters, they used Tampax and I was determined that I would use Tampax. It was a torturous experience trying to learn to put it in because you have to push them very high up otherwise they're sort of on nerves I suppose, and I remember walking around with this Tampax not quite pushed in high enough [laughs] and once I got on to them life was so much better'.[28]

Managing menarcheal and menstrual blood flow for these young girls was clearly problematic in several ways. First, the issue of access to materials, partly determined by income and varying from old rags, cloth or paper for the very poor, to the purchase of suitable absorbent fabric for pad making in more affluent families, to commercially made disposable pads for those with sufficient money who lived in areas of retail distribution. Second, the way in which these devices could be kept in place – the belts, strips of material, loops and pins described and, in the case of a tampon, the difficulty of learning how to place it correctly. Finally, there was the problem of the blood-soaked material and whether to discard it among the household rubbish, or wash and dry it on the family line – both ways introducing issues of privacy. Although many women today can look back and be grateful for advancement in the so-called sanitary hygiene industry, the very different experiences of women from other cultures provide a good framework for looking at the development of that industry.

The issue of access to menstrual absorbents created one of the earliest problems for young immigrant women in transit to Australia – 100 years before my informants made their journeys – and we know about it because of a letter written at the time, significant because so little documentation on the subject of menstruation that has been recovered. A dispatch sent by the vessel's surgeon-superintendent, Dr Richard Eades, to Stephen Walcott, secretary to the organisation responsible for chartering and provisioning the ship, reported inadequate supplies for the immigrant vessel *Roman Emperor*, which had just completed a voyage to Adelaide. The ship carried 221 young women, victims of the Irish famine, for whom regular meals during the voyage were to have unexpected consequences. On arrival in 1848, their plight was reported by Eades in an effort to ensure menstrual towels would be provided on future similar vessels – as much, it seems, for the benefit of young women as for the benefit of others, such as the male crewmembers

---

28   Marjorie, 12, England 1956.

who might witness evidence of the young women's condition by their stained clothing. Concealment of the menstrual condition was required and Eades' demand carries the authority of the male medical establishment:

> I would like to call attention to a matter of hygienic importance viz the total want of cloths or towels among the young females, the majority had not experienced the catamenial flux, which appeared for the first time with more than one half during the voyage, and for which they were unprepared, the perplexity was increased by the difficulty of having the stained linen both of dresses and bedding privately washed. Suitable means should be adopted for this purpose in vessels bringing young females.[29]

Eades' letter points clearly to the social hardship and discomfort menstruating women endured while travelling, in this case for reasons beyond their control. But it also provides medical evidence of the connection between diet and onset of menarche for girls living in conditions of famine.

The difficulties menarche presented for these young 19th-century immigrant women during passage to the Colonies are not without relevance to the memories of my interviewees. Their accounts provide evidence that changes to traditional methods of absorbing menstrual flow were slow and globally uneven, and remain so today. We learned how various sorts of fabrics were folded or sewn as external menstrual absorbents, how pieces of plastic were incorporated by girls in Hong Kong and Vietnam in the 1960s and how the pads were either discarded or washed and reused. But we did not hear of any young girls making tampons and we might ask why, although data suggests the answer is a cultural importance placed on virginity until marriage (and the associated belief that hymenal integrity was proof of virginity). As we learn how extreme deprivation caused some Indian women to remain publicly immobile, squatting on sacks for the duration of their menstrual flow, and how others folded or crushed paper in readiness for the next period, we might ask what the situation is today. Hearing that the onset of a period during a mixed-gender social outing caused shame and fear for the young woman concerned, we might consider how young women in many countries today try to save pieces of absorbent material to hold their menstrual flow, surely an endeavour that is part of the history of women long pre-dating the biblical reference to the 'menstruous cloth'

---

29   Letter, Surgeon-Superintendent Richard Eades, *Roman Emperor,* to the Secretary, Colonial Land and Emigration Commissioners, Stephen Walcott, 25 October 1848, GRG 24/6/1763/1848, State Records of South Australia.

and may traditionally reflect the ecology of an area, for instance shredded bark, moss or animal skin.[30] In 17th-century England shorn wool, or herbs in linen or silk bags, were prescribed as pads or pessaries in conditions of too much or too little menstrual flow, according to Patricia Crawford in her study of attitudes to menstruation at that time. As tampons, these materials were deemed fit for married women so long as they had some sort of thread attachment for removal.[31]

How did the evolution from women's use of primitive materials as menstrual absorbents to the ease of obtaining products developed and manufactured specifically for the purpose come about? This chapter will explore the transition of menstruating women from their confined, domestic and private world into the public sphere. We will examine how Western medical science, technology and marketing created what is now a major international industry based on the concealment of menstruation, while simultaneously revealing its existence through public advertising. Several aspects will be explored, addressing the following questions: what was the social context in which the first manufactured pads were produced and which women benefited most from the innovation? Did women have any input in designs of menstrual absorbents? What benefits did women gain from the technological advances made in menstrual absorbents and how different were the experiences to those who had always used them from the women interviewed who previously had no access to the manufactured product?

The social context from which the early prototypes of modern menstrual absorbents developed will be discussed through events occurring in England and America during the mid-to-late 19th century. These events are part of a wider social change influenced by science and technology that included a deepening social concern about ways of improving the white 'race'.[32] At the time gynaecology, a developing speciality, tended to pathologise menstruation, its theories reflecting male cultural perceptions about girls and women: what they were, and what they ought to be, according to the

---

30   'Isaiah' 30:22, in *The Holy Bible*, King James version, Cambridge University Press, Cambridge n.d. See also Joan Jacobs Brumberg, '"Something happens to girls": menarche and the emergence of the modern hygiene imperative', *Journal of the History of Sexuality*, vol. 4, no. 1, 1993, f.n. 28, p. 113.

31   Patricia Crawford, 'Attitudes to menstruation in seventeenth-century England', *Past and Present*, vol. 91, no. 1, 1981, p. 55. The difference between vaginal tampons and pessaries is the medication contained in the latter.

32   Patricia Vertinsky, 'Exercise, physical capability, and the eternally wounded woman in late nineteenth century North America', *Journal of Sport History*, vol. 14, no. 1, 1987, p. 16.

historian Carroll Smith-Rosenberg.[33] Furthermore, the medical link between menarche, menstruation and disease had expanded to a connection between disease and femininity, made worse by mothers lacking the language for communication with their daughters, as historian Julie-Marie Strange points out.[34] In her study of Victorian women and madness, Elaine Showalter identifies the domestic conditions in which girls experienced pubescence as the basis of emotional vulnerability. This was a time of physical separation from childhood relationships, when many of the daughters of the English upper and growing middle-class saw their brothers off to boarding school. Puberty for boys represented the dawn of male virility and intellectual power but for their sisters, once their companions in all forms of children's activities, it signalled rigid domestic confinement. Girls were privately tutored at home, their education considered secondary to learning the social and domestic arts in readiness for their destiny of marriage. It was a time in which sexual innocence was mandatory until the wedding, and both prudery and ignorance of bodily function prevented many mothers adequately preparing their daughters for menstruation. Consequently, for scores of girls, struggling to manage their periods in households where menstruation had no acknowledged existence, menarche was a shocking experience that, for some, became associated with physical and psychological instability.[35] Although this was inarguably a traumatic time for girls, it should be understood that ignorance about menarche was not specific to the West, as we saw in chapter two. The difference is that in non-industrialised cultures menarche introduced girls to the sexualised world of women through the knowledge and support of their older female kin.

Toward the close of the 19th century, the publication of women's health manuals advised middle-class mothers in America, England and Australia how they might guide their daughters through puberty and menarche. Julie-Marie Strange, writing on teaching menstrual etiquette in England, observes that the promulgation of such knowledge as woman-specific underlines the social taboo surrounding the subject of menstruation.[36] Concealment of menstruation was of prime importance, and some manuals provided patterns for making linen pads, considered superior to cotton,

---

33   Carroll Smith-Rosenberg, 'Puberty to menopause: the cycle of femininity in nineteenth-century America', *Feminist Studies*, vol. 1, no. 3/4, 1973, pp. 60–62.
34   Julie-Marie Strange, 'Teaching menstrual etiquette in England, c. 1920s to 1960s', *Social History of Medicine*, vol. 14, no. 2, 2001, pp. 249–251.
35   Elaine Showalter, *The Female Malady: Women, Madness, and English Culture, 1830–1980*, Penguin Books, New York 1987, pp. 56–57.
36   Strange (2001), p. 252.

which the historian Patricia Crawford suggests is due to the ancient belief that clean linen draws forth moisture. The manuals also advised pre-wash soaking of soiled items. Joan Jacobs Brumberg, in her study on the evolution of American hygiene authority and menarche, argues that although disposable pads began to be manufactured around 1890, those home made from cheesecloth, gauze or left-over dressmaking fabrics were preferred, possibly for reasons of cost, but thoughts about perceptions of cleanliness of manufacture ought also to be considered. The influence of Lister and his theory of antisepsis and the connection between dirt, germs and disease was particularly applicable to women and menstrual blood, and doctors, writing in women's health manuals, emphasised bodily cleanliness during menstruation, including the genital area, and the need for morning and evening pad changes.[37]

Having theorised that menarche and menstruation for girls was a health problem, doctors set about solving it, basing their recommendations on the conviction that women's bodies had finite energy that, in the pubescent girl, must be saved for the optimal development of their reproductive organs. Medical thought had been influenced by the work of Victorian biologist and philosopher Herbert Spencer (1862), who argued that 'Nature was a strict accountant' meeting excessive demands of energy by one part of the body through deprivation elsewhere. Meanwhile biologist Charles Darwin (1874) developed the theme of intellectual difference between men and women, asserting that puberty affected the mental facilities of girls, leaving them, as women, intellectually inferior to men. Somewhat later, psychiatrist Henry Maudsley (1884), pursued Spencer's earlier argument, adding that proper establishment of the female reproductive system drew heavily on vital energies at menarche, so that additional demand, caused by education for example, further depleted reserves of energy leaving some girls vulnerable to disease.[38] It was understood that girls, biologically inferior to their male counterparts, were at risk from the additional stresses placed upon them at puberty. In her article on Victorian-American thoughts on puberty, Smith-Rosenberg points out that not all medical practitioners agreed on the extent

---

37 Brumberg (1993), p. 112–114. See also Crawford (1981), p. 55, f.n. 41.
38 Herbert Spencer, *Education: Intellectual, Moral, and Physical*, Hurst and Company Publishers, New York, 1862, pp. 292–293, http:// www.archive.org/stream/ educationintelle00spenuoft#page/n297/mode/2up; Charles R. Darwin, *The Descent of Man*, second edition revised and augmented, John Murray, London 1874, pp. 564–565, http://darwin-online.org.uk/contents.html#descent; Henry Maudsley, *Sex in Mind and in Education*, C.W. Bardeen Publisher, Syracuse 1884, p. 5, http://www. archive.org/stream/sexinmindandine00maudgoog#page/n8/mode1up

to which limitations should be placed on the activities of the menarcheal girl, although most warned about the hazards of them of becoming too absorbed in any project. Moderate exercise, an almost invalid diet of plain food, and avoidance of stimulating drinks or alcohol were advised. Smith-Rosenberg argues that medical ideas about menarche served social and medical purposes, including an awareness of the development of women's fundamental sexuality, while controlling it within the framework of marriage and maternity. The normality of adolescent emotions and sexuality was accepted with reservation, but preventative medicine for future physiological and psychological health was practised in the form of confinement to the home and limiting activities to the domestic. The alternative – dances, parties, flirting and emotional excitement – were believed to cause madness and disease, including sterility, a belief Smith-Rosenberg attributes to unresolved historical ideas concerning menarche and menstruation.[39]

It is clear that for many young women, particularly those of the more privileged classes, limitations on individual freedoms put in place by medical men (and supported by mothers) kept the problems of menarche in the province of medicine. That was until 1872 when Edward Clarke, a physician and professor of Materia Medica at Harvard Medical School, addressed the New-England Women's Club in Boston.[40] His subject, the relationship between gender and education, caused considerable interest among the wider public and was reported in a number of non-medical journals. In response to this, Clarke decided to enlarge the theme and *Sex in Education; or, a Fair Chance for the Girls* was published in October 1873, with a second edition published the following month, indicating the considerable interest in the topic. Clarke's work came at a time of educational reform in America, when women's political activism for advancement influenced girls' schools to adopt curricula mirroring those of boys. He excluded young working-class women from his concerns, arguing their work-induced physical activities strengthened their bodies and reproductive systems while making their brains torpid, thus ineducable.[41]

Clarke focuses on what he perceives to be the problem of young women in their mid-teens at a time when the age of menarche was most commonly

39   Smith-Rosenberg, (1973), pp. 62–63.
40   Sharra L. Vostral, *Under Wraps: a History of Menstrual Hygiene Technology,* Lexington Books, Lanham, Maryland, 2008, pp. 26–27.
41   Edward H. Clarke, *Sex in Education; or, a Fair Chance for the Girls* (1873), James R. Osgood and Company, Boston, 1875. Project Gutenberg Literary Archive Foundation 2006, pp. 29–30. http:// www.gutenberg.org/ebooks/18504

cited at 14 to 16. He argues that the unhealthy appearance of American girls, compared with their European equivalent, was due to the educational system although the 'perpetual pie and dough-nut' diet, corsets, 'the artificial deformity' of dress, and gynaecological abnormalities all contributed.[42] The core of Clarke's thesis is twofold: the psychophysical problem of girls' educational process causing irregularities in the newly commenced menstrual cycle and the ensuing social problem of sterility leading to the spectre of America being propagated by 'inferior classes'. Clarke argues that the intellectual and muscular effort of study, combined with nervous excitement, deprives the reproductive system of nutrients, which are instead channelled to the brain, an argument not dissimilar to that of Chinese physician Sun Simiao (561–662 CE), referred to in chapter one, who believed that thinking damages the vital organs of a young woman's body.[43] With reference to an earlier work by English psychiatrist Henry Maudsley, Clarke examined clinical aspects of menstrual irregularities, using as evidence examples of high-achieving young women students who became physical and psychological tragedies.[44] Having identified the cause and effect of the problem, Clarke proposed the solution of restructuring the identical co-educational schools, which were based around the needs of boys, to accommodate the needs of girls in the 14 to 18 age group.[45] He recommends that because of their physiological changes girls should have less than eight hours total study time per day, with a recess free from compulsory exercise, and a one to four-day break without penalty, to coincide with menstruation, every fourth week. Clarke refers to England's recent parliamentary passage of the Ten-Hour Act (1875) as a means of women's protection from labour exploitation, although his study excludes any reference to working-class women and adds that the Ten-Hour Act was a recognition of gender difference rather than acknowledgement of women's menstrual cycle.[46]

It comes as somewhat of a relief to read Clarke's clarification that not all young women's gynaecological problems were due to their education, nor that all young graduates were 'pathological specimens'.[47] However, *Sex in*

---

42 Clarke (2006), p. 6.
43 Clarke (2006), pp. 11, 31. See also Sun Simiao, *Prescriptions Worth a Thousand, (Beiji qianjin yaofang)*, cited in Charlotte Furth, *A Flourishing Yin: Gender in Chinese Medical History, 960–1665*, University of California Press, Berkeley, 1999, p. 71.
44 Clarke (2006), pp. 9, 11, 16–24, 27. Henry Maudsley's *Body and Mind* was published in 1870.
45 Clarke (2006), p. 28.
46 Clarke (2006), pp. 34–35.
47 Clarke (2006), p. 26.

Education caused consternation among readers, including Martha Carey Thomas, the American educationalist and president of the American women's college Bryn Mawr, who recalled initial uncertainty about the effect of education on young women's health. Carey Thomas insisted her mother read *Sex in Education*, and was encouraged to learn her mother had never seen, or known of, any young women such as those described by Clarke and thought the whole matter best ignored.[48] *Sex in Education* was reviewed anonymously in the prestigious English medical journal *Lancet* as handling a delicate subject well, without demeaning the intelligence of women, but proving that the handicap of her 'periodic functions' means that to be equal to, she must be more than man. More concisely, as Strange observes, Clarke had constructed a model whereby gender prejudice could be shifted to the physiological.[49]

In England, Clarke's theme was taken up by the 'precociously brilliant, caustic individualist', Dr Henry Maudsley, in the article 'Sex in mind and education', published in the *Fortnightly Review* in 1874.[50] An immediate response to both Clarke and Maudsley by Dr Elizabeth Garrett Anderson was published in the *Fortnightly Review*, bringing the voice of an educated woman to the public. Anderson had resisted the constraints of middle-class life for girls and had been encouraged by her father to gain an education. She commenced training as a nurse in 1860, at a time women were not permitted to study medicine, but discovered that the charter prohibiting her entry to medical school did not apply to the Society of Apothecaries. Consequently, Anderson undertook a five-year apprenticeship to a physician, passing the required examination and becoming a licentiate of the Society. The following year, 1866, she became registered to practise medicine in England.[51] Anderson brings her own experience, and that of many other women, to 'Sex in mind and education: a reply'. This is an important article because although it shows the contrast between the education of girls in America with those in England, and indicates reforms in girls' secondary schooling, as well as the shift in social thought towards higher education

---

48   Elaine and English Showalter, 'Victorian women and menstruation', in *Suffer and be Still: Women in the Victorian Age* (1972), Martha Vicinus (ed.), Indiana University Press, Bloomington, 1973, pp. 41-42.
49   Author undisclosed, 'Reviews and notices of books', *Lancet*, vol. 103, issue 2645, 9 May 1874, p. 661. See also Strange (2001), p. 253.
50   Showalter (1987), pp. 112, 124.
51   Nathan Roth, 'The personalities of two pioneer medical women: Elizabeth Blackwell and Elizabeth Garrett Anderson', *Bulletin of the New York Academy of Medicine*, vol. 47, no. 1, 1971, pp. 71–72.

for women in England, Anderson in effect agrees with Clark that certain allowances for girls at menarche are well justified.

Elizabeth Garrett Anderson begins her critique by expressing her belief that a literary journal was not the appropriate forum for discussing medical and physiological matters, but the need to repudiate both Clarke and Maudsley's arguments that women's education and careers were incompatible with their biology overrode her sense that matters such as this ought to be discussed elsewhere.[52] Anderson observes that menstruation in adult women rarely interferes with normal activities of mind or body beyond a fleeting malaise for a few days, and that poor and working-class women spend all their energies on their labour, without any menstrual rest allowance, and with no known repercussion to their health.[53] However, menarche produces other symptoms, and Anderson considers it to be a time of potentially excessive tiredness and weakness due to accelerated growth, which is dependent on good nutrition, and she recommends some allowances be made by sensible parents or teachers.[54] She challenges Clarke's argument about the psychophysical perils to girls caused by education, and draws attention to the English system, which had already embraced the changes recommended by Clarke. Anderson points out that girls in America take on the stresses of higher education at the age of menarche, and they graduate at 18, studying through the years that Clarke argues to be those of the problematic nervous excitement. In comparison, in England, the regulations at Girton, the girls' college at Cambridge University, prohibit admission before the age of 18, with graduation three or more years later, by which time any nervous excitement of menarcheal change has settled.[55]

Contrasting with the American education system was the reform agenda introduced by the London Association of Schoolmistresses, to promote higher education for girls. School terms were shortened and entrance examinations to Oxford and Cambridge Universities began to be shared. The Association introduced hygiene programs, intended to improve health and vigour, including a daily bath and physical activities such as games and gymnastics. Girls were no longer permitted to stand, reciting, for over an hour at a time, or to sit without proper back support. Their hours of

---

52 Anderson, Elizabeth Garrett, 'Sex in mind and education: a reply', *Fortnightly Review*, vol. 15, no. 89, 1 May 1874, p. 582.
53 Anderson (1874), p. 585.
54 Anderson (1874), p. 586.
55 Anderson (1874), pp. 592–593.

mental work, which included music and needlework, were reduced to six to allow time for play, based on current thought that good results could not be obtained by the sacrifice of one part of the human organism to better another.[56] However, Anderson's most cogent counter-argument to Clarke is that education powers the female mind as good food strengthens the body, and the menstrual cycle does not prevent attainment of this power. Moreover, the psychophysical benefit of an education and career for a woman not only results in her better health but also advantages her children.[57]

While reforms in young women's educational opportunities were being introduced, the conditions for girls among the working poor were also coming under scrutiny. By 1891 in New South Wales, over 40 per cent of women aged 15–24 were employed, 3 per cent of them girls aged 5–14, and the long hours worked by many 'forced to stand all day behind the counters' or 'sweated by clothing factories, and boot factories' had been noted with concern by the social activist William Lane in 1888.[58] However, in America in 1875, following the publication of Clarke's *Sex in Education*, the mills and factories employing women and children working up to 16 hours a day had attracted the attention of Dr Azel Ames, Commissioner of Investigation for the Massachusetts Bureau of Statistics of Labor. Ames interviewed women employed in various industries in an attempt to identify the effects of both work and its conditions on the menstrual function of girls aged 10 to 15, with the object of having child labour practices amended. He argued that poor health in these young women, who lacked financial support, had a social cost and he recommended a periodic rest time of three days a month without penalty to reverse the existing situation of reproductive degeneracy. In her work on the politics of menstruation, historian Sharra Vostral argues that Ames' good intention created problems for working women through his assertion that rest was essential for good reproductive life to benefit the nation. The argument helped influence a court decision in 1908 restricting the employment of women in factories using machinery to 10 hours a day, which Delaney et al argues established state interest in the reproductive bodies of women.[59]

56 Anderson (1874), pp. 587, 593.
57 Anderson (1874), pp. 584, 591–592.
58 Radical socialist William Lane cited in Anne Summers, *Damned Whores and God's Police*, second revised edition, Penguin Books, Camberwell 2002, pp. 355–356.
59 Vostral (2008), pp. 30–31. See also Janice Delaney, Mary Jane Lupton, and Emily Toth, *The Curse: a Cultural History of Menstruation*, (1976), revised edition, University of Illinois Press, Urbana 1988, pp. 55–57.

As we have seen, the reproductive body, specifically the menstruating body, received considerable attention in the late 19th century. Concurrent with the politics of women's education was the work of Lister and the changes in living that followed. In his study of personal hygiene, Andrew Wear points out how the meaning of hygiene shifted from that of health to that of social cleanliness embracing the personal, moral and racial.[60] Cleanliness of person symbolised an inner moral cleanliness, hence 'cleanliness is next to godliness' and, as we saw, the daily bath for girls introduced as part of their education. The importance of personal cleanliness created additional concern about concealment of menstruation, and the stigma any obvious bloodstain would create. Drawers were not worn by English women before the 1840s, and then only by the affluent, as Alia Al-Khalidi showed in her study on menstrual paraphernalia.[61] For poor women, already stigmatised by belonging to 'the great unwashed', change by improvements to living conditions was slow and, as historian Janet McCalman showed in her study of women's health in Melbourne, in the mid-19th century not all women wore undergarments and many impoverished women still menstruated in their clothes. However, in Melbourne, the problems for working-class women remained silenced and hidden by custom in the slums of North Melbourne and Richmond as late as the 1930s. Washing facilities were often a shared outdoor tap, and rags were so special that a household of menstruating women might have only one to share. For these women cleanliness was almost impossible.[62]

Behind the politics of social change in thought and ideas about women and menstruation, a nascent industry was forming, as Alia Al-Khalidi so aptly showed in her study of 19th-century menstrual paraphernalia in Britain. Women's interest in adopting below-knee drawers, or the American bloomer, introduced at the end of the 1840s, and the subsequent outcry against what was considered male dress despite being hidden under petticoats and skirts, focused attention on the pelvic area of the female body and its natural processes.[63] Al-Khalidi argues that this controversy became part of the growing awareness of menstrual matters which ultimately

60   Andrew Wear, 'The history of personal hygiene', in *Companion Encyclopedia of the History of Medicine*, vol. 2, W.F. Bynum and Roy Porter (eds), Routledge, London 1997, pp. 1302–1303.

61   Alia Al-Khalidi, 'Emergent technologies in menstrual paraphernalia in mid-nineteenth-century Britain', *Journal of Design History*, vol. 14, no. 4, 2001, p. 259.

62   Janet McCalman, *Sex and Suffering: Women's Health and a Women's Hospital*, Melbourne University Press, Melbourne, 1998, pp. 18, 180.

63   Al-Khalidid (2001), p. 258–259.

developed into the commodification of menstruation. One outcome was the registering of menstruation-specific technical design patents by British, American and European inventors during the mid-19th century, although as Al-Khalidi noted, registration did not mean the designs were actually manufactured and distributed. However, we can show that specifications and sketches of appliances to be patented in London were indeed precursors to later sanitary hygiene industries, as well as evidence that a sense of thought about the menstrual experience existed. Some patents, utilising recently introduced rubber as moisture-proof rubberised fabric, and elastic, focused on securing an absorbent, rather than on simply being absorbent. They included a design by Theresa Lawrence (1849) of a constructed sanitary belt of red and blue silk with an adjustable piece of elastic in the front, and side insets of soft chamois leather padding, which were repeated under the toggle-type menstrual towel fastener to avoid chafing. Lemuel Dow Owen (1859) registered a menstrual truss using rubber straps, attached to a waistband, to hold two crescent-shaped, air-filled, rubber cushions gripping a sponge or other washable absorbent, covering the labial area. Patent agent William Edward Gedge (1864) applied for registration of a 'catamenial appliance' of form fitting linen-covered silk or oilcloth, with an elastic waistband, and open sides with two deerskin strips attached by buttons each side at both waist level and thigh, holding in place a sponge absorbent, allowing change, or voiding of urine, without the need to remove the whole garment.[64] This form of innovation indicates that securing menstrual absorbents was of major concern for women, but it also indicates that mature women's bodies were the objects of design. There was little suitability in the designs for young menarcheal girls, reflecting Victorian unease about the event.

For young women the problems of menstrual absorbents – their tendency to leak and chafe, and the task of soaking and washing – kept the nuisance aspect of menstruation constantly in mind. In the late 19th century, the development of wood-based absorbents introduced the dimension of dis-posability. According to the journalist Sophia Moseley, an early example was a pad of combined moss and wood shavings developed about 1890 by German naturopath Friedrich Eduard Bliz, which he promoted in his book, *The New Natural Healing*, as having the qualities of being a deodorant, disposable

---

64   Al-Kahlali (2001), pp. 260, 261–264, 272 f.n. 42. Gedge is frequently listed in Chronological Index of Patents Applied and Patents Granted 1863, htpp://www. archive.org/details.chronologicalin05offigoog. As yet there is no 1864 index available online.

and economical to produce.[65] Wood wool was found to have greater powers of absorbency than cotton; among the first commercially manufactured were Hartmann's 'hygienic wood wool towelettes', advertised in Harrod's of London's 1895 catalogue and later reappearing in the end-pages of a midwifery textbook promoting their 'Invaluable and Indispensable' qualities for 'Home Use, Delicate Health, for Ladies Travelling and Accouchement ... After Use they are simply Burnt'.[66] The transition from obstetrical dressing to menstrual pad seems a natural progression and one might ask if the slow acceptance by women was due to cost, the possible odour of antiseptic-impregnated wool, the social embargo on discussion of menstrual matters preventing women's promotion of the product to each other, or the disposal of used pads. 'Simply' burning, as Hartmann's advised, is achieved without fuss in a hospital setting but in the home, disposal of a used pad in the family fire or wood-burning stove entails obvious difficulties. A lack of acceptance was supported by the failure of Johnson and Johnson's initial foray into the American market in 1896 with their disposable Lister's Towels, sold among household sundries in Sears, Roebuck and Company's catalogue. The pads, made from gauze-covered cotton wool with a name denoting the safety and modernity of medical antisepsis, were largely ignored. Delaney et al argue this was because 19th-century morality prevented wide-reaching advertising, but Vostral claims that at the time women could make better pads than they could buy.[67]

Here, as in a number of other areas, the contingencies of war led to new technological developments, in this case the emergence of the absorbent pad. A shortage of cotton for the manufacture of surgical dressings during World War I led to Ernest Mahler, a chemist for the Kimberly-Clark Paper Company of Wisconsin, working on a substitute derived from wood fibre, a cellulose wadding known as 'cellucotton'. This substance was five times more absorbent than cotton, a factor appreciated by Red Cross nurses at the

---

65   Sophia Moseley, 'Practical protection', *Nursing Standard*, vol. 23, no. 6, 2008, pp. 24–25. The type of moss is unidentified but Moseley draws attention to sphagnum moss holding 20 times its dry weight in water.

66   Advertisement for improved obstetric requirements, end-pages, Watson, J. K., *A Complete Handbook of Midwifery for Midwives and Nurses*, The Scientific Press Limited, London, 1904.

67   Delaney et al (1988), pp. 138–139; Irene Heywood Jones, 'Menstruation: the history of sanitary protection', *Nursing Times*, March 1980, p. 407; see also Moseley (2008), pp. 24–25 and Fred E. H. Schroeder, 'Feminine hygiene, fashion and the emancipation of American women', *American Studies*, vol. 17, no. 2, 1976, p. 107. See also Vostral (2008), p.64.

front, who made use of the dressings for their menstrual needs.[68] At the end of the war, left with surplus dressings and aware of their alternative use by the nurses, Kimberly-Clark decided to diversify by forming the Cellucotton Products Company to manufacture disposable menstrual pads. The product would be called Kotex, an amalgam of COtton-TEXture, and sophisticated marketing of the product, beginning in 1921, made it a household name.[69]

This time, in spite of each pad costing 10 cents, there was considerable consumer response among wealthier women, which the historian Vern Bullough associates with two other developments: a wider incorporation of the indoor toilet in middle-class homes and the the changing fashion in women's clothing style to the shorter skirt.[70] Adding to that were developments in transport and communication, making marketing and distribution of the manufactured product more effective, according to historian Andrew Shail in his study of the economics and waste associated with disposable menstrual products.[71] Yet there were cultural constraints, as the historian Joan Brumberg has pointed out, with many Italian-American women expressing fear of health consequences should any interference with menstrual flow occur.[72]

The success of Kotex compelled Johnson and Johnson to re-think the market and the earlier failure of Lister's Towels. They made use of the developments in industrial psychology by consulting Gilbreth Incorporated to research the menstrual habits of women across a spectrum of predominantly young college students, with a smaller representation of high-school students, and professional and businesswomen across the north-eastern states of America. The choice of Gilbreth Incorporated was interesting, not only because women were given a voice in the design of a commercially made menstrual pad, but because the newly widowed Lilian Gilbreth was one of America's early women professionals (with a background in education and

---

68 The story of nurses using dressings as sanitary pads has become part of the Kotex myth and is told in their booklet *The Story of Menstruation* (1946), Kimberly-Clark Corporation, Lane Cove, NSW, 1953, p. 15.

69 Vostral (2008), p. 65; Moseley (2008), p. 25; Delaney et al (1988), p.139; Jones (1980), p. 407.

70 Vern L. Bullough, 'Technology and female sexuality: some implications', *The Journal of Sex Research*, vol. 16, no. 1, 1980, pp. 67–68.

71 Andrew Shail, '"Although a woman's article": menstruant economics and creative waste', *Body and Society*, vol. 14, no. 4, 2007, p. 79. By the 1930s the cost of menstrual pads had fallen significantly. See also Jane Farrell-Beck and Laura Klosterman Kidd, 'The roles of health professionals in the development and dissemination of women's sanitary products, 1880–1940', *The Journal of the History of Medicine and Allied Sciences*, vol. 51, no. 3, 1996, p. 351 f.n. 148.

72 Brumberg (1993), p. 120. See also Crawford (1981), f.n. 41, p. 55.

a PhD in psychology), a university professor, and full business partner of her husband, Frank, an industrial engineer. Moreover, Lilian had borne 12 children and become something of a celebrity through her son and daughter's biography of the eccentricities of Gilbreth family life (later a successful film, *Cheaper by the Dozen*).[73]

The 1927 survey, based on 1037 returned questionnaires, provides the most comprehensive information of young women's menstrual experiences in the inter-war years. It was noted that girls living at home made their menstrual pads, finding them more comfortable than the manufactured product, but they were more likely to be influenced by older colleagues to use disposable absorbents on entering the workplace or college. Other factors in purchase decisions were location and category of merchandiser – chemist or department store – and gender of salesperson. The survey findings indicated clearly what young women wanted in a menstrual pad: comfort, adequate protection, inconspicuousness, disposability and availability, in that order. They stated the desired tab length for fixing the pad to a belt; they were critical of the quality of gauze covering and wanted it softer, and also strengthened to withstand pins or clips; the absorbent material was to be thicker in the centre of the pad and tapering to the ends; and belts to which the pads were fixed needed to be circular, without fasteners, less noticeable, unadorned and easily washed. Kotex were considered too long, too wide, too thick and too stiff. Questions regarding packaging focused on the size and shape of container, ease of opening, its colour and labelling. Most telling were the figures predicting the consumer market, estimated at 30 million women of ages 13–45, each of whom would use 4,576 pads during her menstrual life (given as 32 years), based on the monthly average of 11 pads per woman.

Gilbreth estimated that if only a third of menstruating women used menstrual pads, the market potential for America alone would be over 45,000,000,000. She advised Johnson and Johnson on effective marketing, recommending they maintain 'Modess' as the trademark name, that they alter the shape and size of their pads, and, surprisingly, that they play down the disposable factor because of the problems of blocked toilets, although instructions for disassembling the pad were enclosed in the box.[74] Johnson and Johnson were successful, expanding production of Modess to other countries including Australia in 1932, accompanied by an active advertising

---

73   Vern L. Bullough, 'Merchandising the sanitary napkin: Lilian Gilbreth's 1927 survey', *Signs*, vol. 10, no. 3, 1985, pp. 616–617. See also Vostral (2008), p. 68.

74   Bullough (1985), pp. 616–619, 620–624. See also Vostral (2008), p. 72.

campaign in women's magazines, with stress on 'style and quality' intended to appeal to the middle-class Australian woman. Women had become accustomed to the disposable menstrual pad, but the fear of menstrual odour remained of concern to many, and the discomfort caused by the chafing of a wet pad meant there were many women who would welcome something less cumbersome.[75]

The development of the menstrual tampon evolved from the use of vaginal absorbents in gynaecology and obstetrics either to stop haemorrhage or as an antiseptic. These varying sized plugs of cotton wool or gauze, with tape or twine attached for removal, were first described by a French physician in 1776 and by German physicians in the 1800s, and were traditionally used by circus performers, dancers and other theatrical performers, but it was not until 1933 that a tampon with a disposable applicator, specifically for absorbing the menstrual flow, was patented in America by E. C. Haas of Denver.[76]

The Haas tampon, marketed as Tampax in 1936, was accompanied by a vigorous advertising campaign. Although women were eager consumers they began to ask medical practitioners about the safety of absorbents worn internally. Lack of medical evidence stimulated a series of studies. Two were undertaken in America with grants from the now International Cellucotton Company. The first, in 1938, examined the efficacy of three types of tampons used by 95 women between 18 and 46 years of age. The results indicated that during the days of heaviest flow tampons were obstructive and, used alone, were ineffective in 81.1 per cent of women, who required an external pad to absorb leakage.[77] The second study, carried out between 1939 and 1942, tested 110 women, aged between 19 and 40 years, for any harmful effects caused by tampon use. The results showed no irritation or infection and no obstruction to menstrual flow, although it was found that 65.5 per cent of subjects required an external pad to prevent leak-through on days of heaviest bleeding.[78] However, in 1943 A.E. Taft linked cotton's fruiting-body spores with the germination of moulds and fungi, pointing out that

---

75   Mary Barton, 'Review of the sanitary appliance with a discussion on intravaginal packs', *British Medical Journal*, vol. 1, no. 4243, 1942, p. 524.

76   Madeline Thornton, 'The use of vaginal tampons for the absorption of menstrual discharges', *American Journal of Obstetrics and Gynaecology*, vol. 46, no. 2, 1943, p. 260. See also Vostral (2008), pp. 75–79.

77   Lloyd Arnold and Marie Hagele, 'Vaginal tamponage for catamenial sanitary protection', *The Journal of the American Medical Association*, vol. 110, no. 11, 1938, pp. 790–792.

78   Thornton (1943), pp. 261–265.

ideal conditions for such germination existed in the warmth and moisture of the vagina, sealed by a tampon in the menstruating body.[79] As we will see, this was later to create significant health problems for young women.

Not to be outdone by Tampax, Johnson and Johnson, having diversified with their Personal Products Corporation, began manufacturing Meds in 1940, having innovatively used X-ray technology to evaluate efficiency of the product. They were advertised in Australia as the choice for respectable, thinking women.[80] Medical doubt about tampon use remained, in addition to questions about morality. The idea of young girls handling their genitalia, even becoming familiar with a region of the body supposedly kept in pristine condition until marriage, caused concern. Tampons were deemed unsuitable for the unmarried woman, a judgement upheld by members of the British medical profession in the name of health and expressed in letters to professional journals, including the following two from women practitioners during the Second World War.

> I have had many inquiries from young patients or their mothers concerning the sanitary tampons which can now be obtained. While agreeing with advertisers that this product is, for a married woman, an advance over more old-fashioned ones, the frequent inquiries prompt me to protest against the indiscriminate sale of such goods to young unmarried girls … It is obvious that the use of a tampon may result in rupture of the hymen; and whether or not we consider that this *per se* is to be deplored, I cannot believe that the use of such articles by young virgins can be anything but psychologically bad. Is it not advisable that at least some warning should be printed on the outside of the packings to the effect that the contents may not be satisfactory for unmarried women?[81]

Three weeks later the *Journal* published further medico-moral concerns:

> Shop keepers inform me that this type, and this type only, are asked for by young girls about the ages of 11, 12, and 13 years, and by young women in general. Careful investigation indicates certain undesirable effects from the use of these products (a) Septic infection due to forgetfulness or the belief that frequent changing is unnecessary.

---

79 Charlotte Oram and Judith Beck, 'The tampon: investigated and challenged', *Women and Health*, vol. 6, no. 3, 1981, p. 107.

80 Vostral (2008), p. 96.

81 M. S. Brander, 'Tampons in menstruation', *British Medical Journal*, vol. 1, no. 4239, 1942, p. 452.

(b) Contusion and soreness of the vaginal and labial mucosa due to forcible efforts at insertion. (c) Undesirable handling of vulval area. Many young girls insert tampons with the aid of a looking glass. The psychological ill effects are obvious. (d) Use of tampons by young unmarried girls as a preventative in conditions of promiscuous intercourse.[82]

Social fear of promiscuity and medical fear of infection and psychological damage are combined with criticism of marketing practice in England during wartime. Meanwhile in America, the Navy made the decision that menstrual pads took up storage space and disposal of them blocked the plumbing. Consequently, wartime nurses were supplied with Tampax. Sales increased proportionately as young women in the defence forces, compelled to change their menstrual practices, remained tampon users, and those on production lines at home were targeted by advertising, assuring them that by using Tampax their productivity and patriotism were enhanced. Underlying the shifts in social attitudes toward menstruation were the strongly driven American public health programs that aimed to reduce worker absenteeism by changing menstrual disability to menstrual ability. Women benefited by labouring longer hours in a wartime economy to help the nation, and the tampon manufacturer increased sales by almost 50 per cent between 1942 and 1943.[83]

In Australia, tampons had been sold during the 1930s and advertised, with an emphasis on comfort and freedom, in *Woman* magazine in 1939. However, the Second World War interrupted availability of the English-manufactured product, and it was not until 1947 that an advertisement in the *Australian Women's Weekly* heralded 'Tampax is back'. Nevertheless, the censure of tampon use for young unmarried girls remained firm until the 1960s.[84]

During the 1970s, increased technological knowledge in the USA enabled the development of new absorbent materials, including a tampon named 'Rely' made from a blend of carboxymethylcellulose (CM-cellulose) combined with polyurethane foam chips that offered complete menstrual absorbency.[85] At a time when young women were increasingly benefiting

---

82   Mary G. Cardwell, 'Tampons in menstruation', *British Medical Journal*, vol.1, no. 4242, 1942, p. 537.
83   Vostral (2008), pp. 77, 108–109.
84   Megan Hicks, http:// www.powerhousemuseum.com.rags/internal_protection.php. See also 'To women who love freedom … Tampax is back', *The Australian Women's Weekly*, 29 March 1947, p. 37.
85   Oram and Beck (1981), pp. 112–113, 119.

from internal menstrual absorbents, a situation occurred, resonant with Taft's earlier warning about the potential of cotton tampons for causing germination of fungi. The development of the new super-absorbent tampon enabled rapid growth of bacteria, in this case *Staphyloccus aureus*, or 'golden staph', a pathogen colonising the bodies of many otherwise healthy people. The outcome varied, with menstruating teenagers most affected by either mild flu-like symptoms, or the more serious sudden onset of fever with diarrhoea and vomiting, dramatic drop in blood pressure, and a rash on the face, hands, and feet described as toxic shock syndrome.[86] Rely was withdrawn by its manufacturers (Procter and Gamble) in September 1980, after 814 clinical cases and 38 deaths had been reported in the USA, and with case reports from other countries including Australia. Nevertheless, other tampons with a similar high-absorbency content remained on the market, each packet carrying a regulation warning about the link with toxic shock syndrome from June 1982.[87] The Rely misadventure is evidence of change both in technological development and in human pathogens and Vostral points out that, as a result, women shunned tampons, choosing safety over the advertised freedom.[88]

Conclusion

The chapter is divided into two distinct parts. The first examines the interview data, which indicates the concern shared by women from diverse cultures over concealment of menstruation from the onset of menarche. The second examines the historic background to the evolution of disposable sanitary hygiene absorbents, now a major international industry.

The data confirms that until the 1960s, women in non-industrialised countries and cultures shared many of the factors that had denied Western women access to menstrual hygiene products in the 1920s–1940s. These included cost, sanitation facilities for disposal, wider geographical distribution and, in the case of tampons, belief in moral and physical damage to girls' bodies. The data also gives an example of the way in which women's clothing, the long sulus, saris, kaftans and hijabs, concealed both the body

---

86   Steven D. Helgerson, 'Toxic-shock syndrome: tampons, toxins, and time: the evolution of understanding an illness', *Women and Health*, vol. 6, no. 3, 1981, pp. 93, 99–100, 102.

87   Nancy J. Cibulka, 'Toxic shock syndrome and other tampon related risks', *The Journal of Obstetric, Gynaecologic and Neonatal Nursing*,vol. 12, no. 2, 1983, pp. 94–97. See also Vostral (2008), p. 157 and Helgerson (1981), p. 101.

88   Vostral (2008), p. 163.

and the menstrual cloths and rags used to absorb menstrual blood. By contrast, Australian advertisements for sanitary hygiene products during the 1930s indicated that clothing was becoming more shaped to the body of women, preceding the adoption of shorter skirts.

Poverty was a major determinant of access to disposable menstrual absorbents in Western countries, as demonstrated by the instance of sisters in an industrial area of Melbourne, without indoor sanitation, who reportedly shared menstrual rags and whose hardship, like that of many others in similar circumstances at the time, remained hidden. Interview data gives similar instances of girls at menarche deprived of pads and having to use rags, paper, or for one young menstruating woman, an Indian squat.

Concealment is part of the long history of ideas about women and their menstruating bodies, becoming increasingly significant because of social change in the late 19th century. Part of this change affected women through their greater entry into the public space via access to higher education and employment. As women entered the public sphere, controlling and concealing menstruation became increasingly important and difficult to practise through traditional means, so what had historically been a women's matter moved into the realm of men. Medical advancement demonstrated the links between pathology and hygiene, resulting in scientific research developing disposable surgical dressing materials with properties for greater absorbency. The establishment of the sanitary hygiene industry followed and the role played by women in the early development of disposable menstrual absorbents was discussed.

Concealing menstruation continued to grow easier as women increasingly gained access to disposable sanitary hygiene products while, paradoxically, newspaper and magazine advertisements for the products kept the existence of menarche and menstruation publicly visible. Although the rhetoric of freedom through concealment continued to be part of menstrual product promotion in industrialised countries, it reinforced the perception that menstruation is both disabling and visibly shameful. Moreover, women consumers remained vulnerable, as the introduction of super-absorbents in tampons proved, indicating that innovation in sanitary hygiene products can have serious consequences.

Chapter 7

WHAT *SHOULD* EVERY YOUNG GIRL KNOW?

Kotex sent people into our school.[1]

'What should girls be permitted to know about menstruation?' This was a question of considerable social concern in early 20th-century Australia because it introduced girls to the knowledge of their bodies and bodily functions. These were topics still widely believed to be unsuitable for young females, leading into the realms of a little knowledge being a dangerous thing, particularly if it stimulated interest in the realm of sexuality. So the risk of endangering young girls who were to be the future mothers of the country resulted in considerations of who should have authority over the knowledge. Was the Australian concern shared in other cultures? What did the women interviewed remember of the cultural attitudes in their native countries? For instance, who should have the responsibility for menstrual education? Mothers? Older women within the family such as aunts or grandmothers? Should the responsibility be with women external to the family such as school teachers? Or even women at all? Should knowledge about menstruation be transmitted from household medical texts written by men? And when should this knowledge be given or allowed to be accessed? How soon before menarche? Or not until menstruation occurs?

Although the shifts in thought affecting how Australian girls learned about menarche and menstruation had little relevance to girls in other cultures at the time, they had a later significance. Consequently, in this chapter I will consider three issues: the ways in which interviewees remembered learning about menarche and menstruation and their channels of information; the changing ways in which Australian girls' sources of information moved from maternal authority in the privacy of the home

---

1   Sue, 13 years old at menarche, Singapore 1967.

to increasingly public knowledge influenced by religious and medical philosophy; and the appropriation of the role of teacher by sanitary hygiene manufacturers. This will be discussed through the chronological progression of product advertisements for each of the two major companies from the 1930s to the 1950s in their construction of the menstruating woman. This third issue is relevant to the interviewees because they influenced Australian women's social attitudes toward menarche and menstruation, and this culture was encountered by immigrant women and girls in the workplace, labour ward, schoolyard and classroom, as they moved through their daily lives in what was often, for them, a unilateral experience.

Cultural attitudes toward pre-menarcheal knowledge of menstruation determined the way in which the interviewees acquired knowledge. Sun was at a Christian school in Korea, a country described by her compatriot, Jung, as 'not open to woman'. Sun recalled 'I knew a little bit at the time. The school had been teaching me'.[2] Cecile stated simply, 'in our culture it is not said' and Ruth remembered 'my mum had not talked to me about this at all'.[3] Keshini remained perplexed that her 'mother had never, never, discussed this with me' and Rosalia conveyed the resentment of being kept in ignorance: 'Mama never told me anything'.[4] This was echoed by Wani – 'my mother didn't tell me anything about what menstruation was' – and by Marjorie, who recalled that 'no one had actually discussed this with me within the family'.[5] Virisila commented that 'even though my mum was a midwife we never discussed menstruation' a cultural issue confirmed by Levani: 'you don't talk to your mother about these things'.[6] There was bitterness in Alisha's memories: 'they never told us anything. They didn't guide us. That sort of education is not given to girls, so they're ignorant'.[7]

Yet others such as Rashida had learned in advance from their mothers – 'she tell me before' – and Karuna remembered 'my mother told me when I was young'.[8] Karuna's preparation was repeated by Seda. 'I know about it because my mother explained to me two years before'. She added 'I had no grandmothers at this time but now I become grandmother I explained about it because my daughter said "I am ashamed, Mama, do it for me,

2   Sun, 13, South Korea 1962; Jung, 13, South Korea 1959.
3   Cecile, Uganda 1965; Ruth, 17, Uganda c.1974.
4   Keshini, 12, Sri Lanka 1969; Rosalia, 13, Italy 1950.
5   Wani, 13, Indonesia 1954; Marjorie, 12, England 1956.
6   Virisila, 11, Fiji 1964; Levani, 16, Fiji 1967.
7   Alisha, c.14, India c.1943.
8   Rashida, 14, Lebanon, year unknown; Karuna, Kenya, age and year of menarche unknown.

explain your view to your granddaughters'".[9] Cosmina remembered how she 'woke up and asked for Mother. Mother explained everything'.[10] However, Ramona recalled her mother's information being limited to 'look, Ramona you're going to have your period and after that you have to look after yourself because you're going to be a little lady', which told her little about the menstrual process, but much about the Spanish-Chilean importance of maintaining virginity until marriage. Lola was also dissatisfied by her mother's lack of explanation when she reported, 'Mum, I think I've got my period'. Her mother's response was identical to that Ramona received. Lola continued, 'with all this I would like to make a comment. I would wish for more explanation, some more information about what a period is because if it weren't for my sister, the one I saw, what happens if I had two brothers and no sister? That would have been a shock for me one day to find I was bleeding from the vagina'.[11]

Lack of maternal instruction and support was frequently compensated for by friends whose knowledge of science-based physiology was limited, but who provided a forum for exchanging thoughts and concerns in cultures where maternal silence existed. Jung, for, instance, remembered that she heard about menstruation 'from friends who had their periods ... a bit shocked'.[12] Qing recalled that 'only my peer group explained to me what menstruation was' and Levani 'knew all about the period because you talk to your friends'.[13] Elena remembered being confident because 'I know a bit from the friends ... I'm ready'.[14] Nirmala related how her 'mum was always busy trying to make a living, and also my grandma. I have to learn myself, so the first friend who had the period we would ask her what did it feel like? That's how I learnt because in Indonesia, even though you were at school, we don't have sex education like, you know, body'.[15] Verisila recalled that at boarding school 'someone talked about it in passing but I really was not paying attention. I thought OK, I'm too young for this. You know, that's how I felt then'.[16] Hetal, motherless, lived in a large extended family as the eldest girl, but 'nobody said me anything. I was told by friends' and Marjorie reminisced that 'my mother didn't explain anything to me but a girl who

9   Seda, 14, Armenia, year unknown.
10   Cosima, 12, Moldavia 1953; Nirmala, 13, Indonesia 1964.
11   Ramona, 15, Chile 1964; Lola, 17, Chile 1967.
12   Jung, 13, South Korea 1959.
13   Qing, 12, Hong Kong 1962; Levani, 16, Fiji 1967.
14   Elena, 14, Greece, year unknown.
15   Nirmala, 13, Indonesia 1964.
16   Virisila, 11, Fiji 1964.

started her periods in primary school was my sex educationalist. She told me everything and I didn't believe her'.[17]

There were other ways of acquiring knowledge – girls with older sisters and cousins observed, often unconsciously, indications of cyclically different behaviour and hygiene practice, especially noticeable in close living conditions without modern sanitation. Beatriz recalled 'no one explained about your first period' but 'I saw my sister who was a year older and that means I saw how she was having the period'. Lolas's memories were similar. 'I knew what was coming because I saw my sister – my sister was older than me' and Delia, too, 'knew a little bit more because I have an older sister'. Nadia remembered 'hearing my sister talking about it because she's older than me. She was telling my mother about her period so that's how I was a bit aware of it'. Neve related that 'my sister show me and teach me everything, not my mother' and Alcina reflected similarly, 'I know because I have the sisters'.[18] Cecile 'knew what it is and also I'd seen some girls at school'.[19] Corazon had older girl cousins living with her family, and observed with interest how 'every month they have all this. I saw them washing their undies and sometimes I found stains on the clothing or even bedsheets'.[20] Lee believes that, like many girls at the time, she 'was learning by the knowledge of what you see, and what you gather, and what happened to your mum. Folding papers gives you a glimpse'.[21]

A small sample of interviewees had been exposed to the effects of advertising, and this was apparent in their reference to sanitary pads as 'Kotex' or 'Modess', the trade names that came to symbolise far more than simply an absorbent pad, as we shall see. In the Philippines Domini recalled that 'around 1960 when I was first year high school … in physical education … we have time being taught how to use these things and then, sometimes, people from this company, they come to school and give us hygiene education and how to dispose of [used pads]. They show us movies about how this thing happens, the cycles and everything, and teach us'. In answer to the question about whether or not this was helpful Domini's response was immediate: 'very helpful, because I was in first year high school that it [menarche] happened and then every year, up to four, they have a new

---

17   Hetal, 14, India c.1952; Marjorie, 12, England 1956.
18   Beatriz, 12, Chile c.1960; Lola, 17, Chile 1967; Delia, 11, Greece 1960; Nadia, 11, Alexandria 1950; Neve, 11, Italy 1941; Alcina, 15, Italy 1947.
19   Cecile, 16, Uganda 1965.
20   Corazon, 12, Philippines 1956.
21   Lee, 13, Singapore 1962. See previous chapter for reference to folding papers.

product they come to school to talk about'.[22] Sue remembered that product promotion through education had begun in Singapore schools during the 1960s. 'I went to a mission school, a convent, and Kotex, which was like a key brand name in Singapore – there was Kotex, there was Modess, those were the two I knew of – Kotex sent people into our school to sort of talk to the students about it and I remember, aged about twelve or something, I had no idea what they were talking about'.[23]

Domini and Sue were the only two women interviewed who had received menstrual education from a sanitary hygiene company representative at their schools. Domini found it helpful, but Sue was unable to relate to the information at all, a not uncommon situation today according to paediatric researchers Kelly Orringer and Sheila Gahagan, who find such instruction poorly retained.[24] That only 2 of 54 women interviewed had received this form of guidance is understandable in the context that only 12 of the 54 had used commercially made sanitary pads at menarche. The remainder were living in countries, or areas of countries, beyond the reach of manufacture and distribution of the products and the associated forms of advertising. Their knowledge belonged to women and followed traditional paths including restricted maternal preparation for menarche. The cultural silence of mothers was offset by the agency of friends, whose subjective experience-based knowledge allayed anxiety for many girls. The interviews also drew attention to the importance of biological timing on the ability of pubescent girls to understand information about menstruation, and provided the interesting perspective of knowledge acquired through the observation of older menstruating sisters and cousins, allowing adjustment to the idea of becoming a menstruating woman.

From the 1930s Australian mothers had been able to obtain guidance in preparing their daughters for menstruation. The earliest text published by a sanitary hygiene company was *Marjorie May's Twelfth Birthday*, and it was promoted to help 'modern mothers' discuss 'intimate problems with a sensitive, growing daughter'.[25] The free, mail-order booklet, obtainable from Australian Cellucotton Products (the manufacturers of Kotex), remained popular throughout the 1940s. *Marjorie May's Twelfth Birthday*

---

22   Domini, c.13, Philippines 1960.
23   Sue, 13, Singapore 1967.
24   Kelly Orringer and Sheila Gahagan, 'Adolescent girls define menstruation: a multiethnic exploratory study', *Health Care for Women International*, vol. 31, no. 9, 2010, p. 841.
25   Mary Pauline Callender, *Marjorie May's Twelfth Birthday*, Australian Cellucotton Products P/L., Sydney 1932.

is about sanitary hygiene and reflects the historian Joan Jacobs Brumberg's argument that in America from the 1920s, sanitary hygiene was the major focus at menarche, with discussions about menstruation carefully avoiding the danger zones of developing adolescent sexuality, thus desexualising the menarcheal girl.[26] In the 1932 Australian edition, Marjorie May is portrayed as a sensitive little girl in contrast with the more sophisticated adolescents in later publications of the genre.

The text is constructed around an affectionate post-birthday party talk that Marjorie and her mother have, initiated by Marjorie expressing puzzled disappointment that her 'chum' Margaret, a few months older, was reluctant to join in the party games. Marjorie's mother explains that Margaret has begun to menstruate, a process referred to as purification, and that she has successfully concealed it from everyone by using Kotex. Marjorie is delighted to learn of the experience she will soon share and also to hear about, and be shown, the wonderful 'clean looking' pads. She has learned the first lesson about menstruation: that of concealment, which the anthropologist Cathryn Britton argues is a form of individual seclusion transmitted through family, peers, educational organisations and advertisements.[27] Nonetheless, Marjorie is extremely grateful to her mother for telling her the exciting news and comments, 'I will feel quite a young lady when the new purification comes'.

In 1946, following the success of animated films like Snow White and Bambi, Walt Disney was commissioned by Kimberly-Clark's International Cellucotton Productions Company to make a 10-minute educational film, *The Story of Menstruation*.[28] The Second World War had ended and the baby boom was beginning, but this was not a sex-education film and no link was made beyond the nebulous unfertilised egg causing breakdown of the uterine lining and the resultant menstrual flow. Although *The Story of Menstruation* appears quaint today, when viewed in the social context of the time it succeeds as a teaching device, constructed to avoid controversy by not impinging on the maternal right to determine what knowledge would be given to her daughter and by whom. According to the historian

---

26 Joan Jacobs Brumberg, '"Something happens to girls": menarche and the emergence of the modern hygiene imperative', *Journal of the History of Sexuality*, vol. 4, no. 1, 1993, p. 123.

27 Cathryn J. Britton, 'Learning about the 'the curse': an anthropological perspective on experiences of menstruation', *Women's Studies International Forum*, vol. 19, no. 6, 1996, p. 650.

28 Kotex Products, *The Story of Menstruation*, Walt Disney Productions 1946, http://www.youtube.com/watch?v=bjIJZyoKRIg

Sharra Vostral in her study of menstrual hygiene technology, it was used in schools for over 35 years and reached over 105 million women.[29] These young girls from many cultures watched, and possibly internalised, the unfolding of an American woman's life – symbolised by blossoms, blocks, girlie-dolls and books – to the pubescent Snow White look-alike with maturing hormones. The physical process of the menstrual cycle is diagrammatic, simple and clear, with a non-confrontational menstrual flow. Having explained the 'why' of menstruation, the film moves to the 'how' with a mature-voiced, reassuring, woman narrator who advises exercise during menstruation, but avoidance of horse-riding, cycling or lifting heavy weights. 'Snow White' wears a bathing cap in the shower and avoids very hot or very cold water, but readers are told warm baths and showers are essential because of perspiration odour 'on those days'. This information was intended to dispel the residual myths of menstruation perpetuated by the non-modern mother, but still maintains traces of those very myths. The psychological aspect is included with advice about the importance of controlling misery or self-pity, illustrated by a bad-hair day, and that avoiding constipation and having a good diet will help with both. Emotional excitement combined with violent activity is construed as perilous, and we see frenetic jitterbugging with a boyfriend as a likely cause of danger. The ubiquitous 'cramp' or 'twinge' is helped by exercises like toe-touching and by correct posture. Menstrual organisation is stressed, and girls are reminded to mark the date of their next period on the calendar. Looking good while menstruating is emphasised by 'Snow White' smiling at her reflection in the mirror of her powder compact, as the narrator speaks of cycles. We see her as a bride, followed by a baby repeating the opening scene, exemplifying life for a woman in 1946.

The Story of Menstruation has an underlying concern with adolescent behaviour masked by menstrual advice. Bad diets, dance crazes, late nights, risky activities and self-interest are all alluded to without elaboration. This concern was not confined to America. In 1951 Melbourne, the dangers of girls having only limited knowledge about basic bodily processes concerned social groups, including the Federation of Mothers' Clubs, who believed women needed access to accurate information about menstruation and reproduction to enable them to educate their daughters. To that end it

---

29   Sharra Vostral, *Under Wraps: a History of Menstrual Hygiene Technology*, Lexington Books, Lanham, Maryland 2008, pp. 123–124. Brumberg states that *the Story of Menstruation* has been seen by 93 million American women, indicating that it reached 12 million girls outside America. See also Brumberg, (1993), p. 124.

was proposed that the Director of Physical Education at the University of Melbourne, Dr Fritz Duras, who lectured widely on human reproduction, be invited to attend a showing of *The Story of Menstruation* during a conference of the Federation of Mothers' Clubs. At the completion of the film Dr Duras would give a talk to the women in attendance who wished for approval, by the Director of Education, to have the film shown to all secondary school girls in Victoria and to 'all teen-age girls in State schools'.[30] In this the Federation of Mothers' Clubs demonstrated some ambivalence, suggesting that mothers should be the principal educators of menstrual matters while at the same time lobbying the Department of Education to have the information supplied by Kimberly-Clark and others through their films and talks given to girls at school.

In an odd recognition of the other half of the population, the Father and Son Welfare Movement, established in 1926, published *The Guide Through Girlhood*, written by Florence Kenny and edited by Professor Harvey Sutton, principal medical officer for the Department of Education, NSW. The purpose of the 1946 publication, with its male medical authority, was to reinforce the message of special mother and daughter film nights and slide shows, dedicated to educating mothers and girls from eight to twelve years, about the 'problems' of life in a 'clean, wholesome manner'. *The Guide* would also reach mothers and daughters living in more remote areas. The text begins with the role model of Jesus Christ, not unexpected in the Father and Son Movement, but omitting the gender-compatible Virgin Mary with her Roman Catholic connotation. There is an emphasis on how Jesus, at 12 years old, was growing mentally, intellectually, physically, socially and spiritually, all qualities young girls might aspire to, particularly in thoughts about themselves and their pre-pubescent bodies, at a time of post-war idealism about young women's sexual purity.[31]

The Guide Through Girlhood suggests that girls think of their bodies as wonderful and complex machines, with diagrams to assist their understanding of the organs of reproduction and their location. Menstruation is explained as a shedding of the uterine lining, usually every 28 days, with the flow leaving the body through a girl's 'private part', a 19th-century

30 'Showing of sex education films', *The Argus*, 23 February 1951, p. 7. See also reference to Dr Fritz Duras, 'Lack of physiological knowledge held harmful to young people', *The Mercury*, 14 January 1946, p. 9.
31 Florence Kenny, *The Guide Through Girlhood*, Prof. Harvey Sutton (ed.), published by the Father and Son Movement, Sydney 1945, pp. 2–3. This was still in publication in 1961. See also Megan Hicks, 'The rags: paraphernalia of menstruation', http://www.powerhousemuseum.com/rags/advice_for_girls.php

euphemism signalling a topic of silence, so it came as a relief to hear the correct anatomical term, vagina, used in an almost identical explanation in *The Story of Menstruation*. *The Guide* informs mothers and daughters that ignorance of menarche produces fear and dread, often leading to concealment and a further cycle of fear the following month. On discovering their menarche, girls are advised to go immediately to tell their mothers 'or whoever has charge of you'. Brumberg's 'hygiene imperative' is apparent in such a directive, with concealment of stained clothing by a cloth and instructions on how to fasten it being the prime acknowledgement that mother, or carer, can provide.[32] Disposable menstrual absorbents are not mentioned. Reassurance comes through the amazing news that bleeding signals the physical changes that will turn them into women and prepare them to become mothers, news that some may find quite perplexing. Further recommendations of how to manage this 'problem', another unfortunate euphemism, included bathing, and avoidance of both constipation and the use of laxatives, reminding us that in the 1940s laxatives for children were accepted practice for regular bowel habits. However, there were preferred ways, and a good diet of fresh fruit and vegetables and plenty of water to drink are advised. The late 19th-century association between menarche, menstruation and unwellness is dispelled.[33]

Kimberly-Clark's International Cellucotton Products Company's *Very Personally Yours* was published in America in 1946 to reinforce the message of *The Story of Menstruation* and to extend promotion of the manufacturer's product, Kotex sanitary pads. An Australian version was published much later, around 1962, containing minor changes to accommodate idiomatic differences. Whereas the film omitted any reference to sanitary hygiene products, *Very Personally Yours* is an advertising tool in the guise of an educator, linking menarche to an 'exciting' new form of consumerism.[34] Nonetheless, the explanation of menarche as a physical phenomenon is clear, and benefits from being stripped of the euphemisms of *The Guide Through Girlhood*. Both texts reflect the interests of publishers, and of society, with Kimberly-Clark emphasising the material aspect of life, and the Mother and Daughter subsection of the Father and Son Welfare Movement placing stress on moral principles, strong stuff for the targeted age group – work, independence, and responsibility.

---

32   Brumberg, (1993), pp. 100–101.
33   Kenny, (1945), pp. 6–7.
34   *Very Personally Yours*, Education Department for Kimberly-Clark of Australia, Lane Cove, NSW 1962, pp. 2–19.

Menstrual 'unwellness' is derided by both, the Movement arguing effect rather than cause, explaining the added burden for others, both domestically and in the workplace. The Movement girl learns to prepare herself for a life of industrious reliability, in contrast with the Kotex girl who has 'waited on tip-toe for the day of days that would mark the commencement of a wonderful adventure'.

It was not until 1949 that the Australian Cellucotton Products Company released a replacement booklet for the rather dated *Marjorie May*. That Australian text did not replicate the 1940 American version, in which a mother instructed her daughter in matters of menstrual hygiene 'as one girl to another', a situation Vostral argues to have infantilised the mother.[35] The Australian *As One Girl to Another* precedes any acknowledgment of early multiculturalism and is an English-language only text. It deals lightly with several adolescent concerns, beginning with recognition of sexual attraction, changes in physical and behavioural patterns, developing self-realisation, all leading to the menarcheal event which comes as 'a bit of a nuisance' to be resolved by Kotex. Advice about adjusting to the monthly cycle is given with further advice regarding individual differences in cycles. Keeping a menstrual calendar is emphasised, and instruction is given about preparing for the next period and why purchasing Kotex from a young man need not cause embarrassment. Pre-menstrual symptoms such as fluid retention and subsequent weight gain are mentioned, and personal hygiene products are promoted including deodorant talc to be sprinkled on Kotex pads to mask odour as a supplement to bathing. Moderate exercise and enjoyment of a normal social life with friends is recommended for the menstruating girl. The subject of tampons is introduced with caution, and the advice to consult a doctor before use, because of the hymen, is given. It argues that pads are better for young girls and gives diagrammatic instructions of how to fasten a pad to a Kotex sanitary belt.[36]

Not to be outdone, Johnson and Johnson published *Growing Up and Liking It* in the 1950s, obtainable by sending a coupon attached to an advertisement for Modess to Nurse Reid at Johnson and Johnson, thus investing the publication with the authority of the female health professional.[37] The booklet was the first of its kind to be illustrated by photographs of teenage girls enjoying an active heterosexual social life: dancing, clothes shopping, cheering favourite sports teams and wearing their first full-length formal

---

35   Vostral (2008), pp. 120–121.
36   *As One Girl to Another*, Australian Cellucotton Products P/L., Sydney 1949, pp. 1–18.
37   'Free', *Growing Up ... The Mercury*, 22 August 1952, p. 4.

dress. Pre-teens may have difficulty relating to the text, something that would not be helped by the opening paragraph informing them that the experience of menarche is what they have been waiting for. Readers are told it symbolises that they are of an age to think for themselves and gives examples such as choosing their own clothes, noticing boys and being the object of their attention and partaking in a series of 'firsts': first date, first party, first formal dance. The physiological explanation of the menstrual cycle is brief, diagrammatic and less clear than offered in *Very Personally Yours*, with the only reference to Australian girls being their average age of menarche, given as 12. If that was the target age for the text it seems to do less well. It is humourless and probably too sophisticated in its approach to menstrual questions and answers, with old wives' tales, strategies for developing self-confidence about menstruation, do's and don'ts with a certain stress on cosseting the self from the elements, general health advice on diet, appearance and sleep, and a general pattern of exercises for health and well-being appropriate for menstrual cramps. 'Important pointers' are made, including prohibition of flushing a used disposable pad down the toilet, and when to see a doctor. Interestingly both booklets provide two-year calendars for marking menstrual cycles, inferring constant reference will be made during that time, enabling some 'growing into' the texts.[38]

The booklets indicate how the concept of early adolescence was constructed between 1932 and 1962. *The Guide Through Girlhood* blends philosophy through the model of Protestant Christianity adapted to women, science in the anatomical and physiological explanation of menstruation, and the social mores that dictate the use of euphemisms rather than correct terminology for perceived sensitivities of young girls and, possibly, their mothers. It seems most unlikely that girls would seek to obtain their own copy of *The Guide*. Nor was *Marjorie May's Twelfth Birthday* promoted towards girls as consumers. Far from it, given the picture of a distraught looking pre-teenage girl captioned 'Mother dear – I need you *so much!*' One can almost picture Mother running to get her pen, urged by the paragraph below which, surprisingly, refers to menstruation by word in a daily newspaper:

> Don't fail her in her first serious experience. It is so important that your daughter learns the truth from *you first*. Do not wait until it is too late to give her the necessary facts about menstruation. In too many cases, girls are shocked and frightened when this experience comes

---

38   *Growing Up and Liking It* (1952), Johnson and Johnson Pacific Limited, no publishing details, c. 1968, pp. 2–25.

unexpectedly. That is why we urge you to send for the FREE booklets which have helped millions of mothers give their daughters a happy, healthy approach to womanhood.[39]

By the late 1940s girls were constructed as becoming more independent. The advertisement for *As One Girl to Another* is directly addressed to the girl herself. She no longer calls to her mother not to fail her, but acts independently to obtain information about menstruation, in this instance by filling out and mailing a coupon. The caption follows:

Here is a booklet every lass needs, dedicated to Australian girls by Kotex. From it you'll learn about the adventure of growing up … how to manage your social life … how to feel secure and comfortable every day of the month.[40]

Very Personally Yours and *Growing Up and Liking It* continue the association between menarche and growing independence and are similar in content and expression, but with the former inclined to employ the euphemisms, 'certain days' and 'those days' for menstruation, sending a negative message of difference. Although *Growing Up and Liking It* references menstruation as a cause for pride in achieving physical maturity, it uses only material examples, shopping and social activities, to signify coming of age. The text is informative, but lacking the humour that would lighten the message and appeal more to pre-teens, and there are no euphemisms. The commonality in all hygiene product texts is the body as untrustworthy, bleeding – often unexpectedly – cramping, undermining confidence by its tell-tale staining and associated limitations in social and sporting activities. The solution lies in control by becoming a consumer of the manufactured products in a partnership of need and supply.

However, need and supply are situations not exclusive to each other. The young potential consumers, the newly menstruating girls, enjoyed experimenting with the products available to them, causing manufacturers to constantly compete for their custom, and product loyalty, through advertising. The ways in which women are constructed in these advertisements reflect social ideals of the time, telling a story to readers, including young girls whose interest in the products is stimulated by their menarcheal experience and the way in which they perceive the story. I want to show this development during the 1930s to 1950s and particularly the 1939–1945

39   'Mother dear – I need you so much!' *The Mercury*, 30 January 1940, p. 6.
40   'Free', *As One Girl to Another, The Mercury*, 11 March 1949, p. 7.

Second World War years. Australian daily newspapers are my main source, some with dedicated women's supplements, others scattered through the main body of news, and all pictorial representations are commercially drawn in black and white. Although many women did not read newspapers, they did see advertisements as they handled the paper as a domestic or workplace utensil. The second source used is the *Australian Women's Weekly*, which was part of family life during the time.

The early newspaper advertisements placed by the International Cellu-cotton Products Company in 1928 were simply a box of Kotex with a large tick and a warning to women not to be careless about their health, stating categorically that all doctors recommended safe sanitary napkins.[41] At the time medical authority to validate women's sanitary hygiene products was still sought from a disproportionately male profession, with emphasis remaining on the association between good health and disposable menstrual absorbents. A construction of woman as consumer was, as yet, undefined. In 1931 the company announced the establishment of a 'highly efficient' factory to manufacture Kotex in Australia,[42] and the following year Johnson and Johnson announced the availability of Modess as 'women's most intimate personal accessory'. The Modess woman lacks a face but she knows what she wants: a totally disposable, more absorbent and softer filler, and softer gauze, all of which accord with the American Gilbreth findings of 1927, discussed in the previous chapter.[43] A week later we meet the Modess woman. Slender, young but age indeterminate, she is alone, signifying independence. She is seated on a bench outdoors, indicating removal from domestic matters, and she is casually but elegantly dressed in slacks, short-sleeved fitted shirt, and cartwheel sun-hat, denoting her modern outlook.[44] Next time we see her she is short-skirted and bashing a tennis ball – 'she wants freedom and comfort and will not tolerate the drudgeries that held her mother in bondage'.[45] She is an active role model for the menarcheal girl, but the more mature woman was not ignored and a series of sophisticated non-domestic representations followed. This Modess

---

41 'Next time ... Kotex', *The Argus*, 13 April 1928, p. 18.
42 'The establishment of a highly efficient factory', *Sydney Morning Herald*, 20 February 1931, p. 6s.
43 'Announcing women's most intimate personal accessory', *The Brisbane Courier*, 16 February 1932, p. 17.
44 'To meet the requirements of the modern woman', *The Brisbane Courier*, 23 February 1932, p. 17.
45 'To meet the requirements of the modern woman', *The Brisbane Courier*, 1 March 1932, p. 17.

woman is always slender and glamorously dressed, according to fashions of the time, with daytime gloves, heels, hat and bag signifying a leisured existence; at night she is fur-draped in a long form-fitting gown, the text describing 'gracious softness, a yielding pliancy' in a deliberately ambiguous product description.[46]

Advertisements for Australian Cellucotton Products, manufacturers of Kotex, were far less ambiguous. They relied on text to undermine the competition through fear tactics, asking 'How about the nameless substitutes? How are they made? Where? By whom? How do you know they're fit for intimate use?'[47] Their newspaper advertisements continued as a brief text alongside an illustration of the product until 1941, by which time Australia was at war and the Kotex woman was introduced. She is dancing romantically, her partner in a white tuxedo, and she wears a short-sleeved jacket over a long full skirt. She symbolises 'the poise of confidence. Lilting music ... exciting people. You want to live every minute. There's no time or place for self-conscious discomfort or worry'.[48] There is a sense of impending separation from partners and, indeed, familiar life, but for the younger Kotex woman life is full of promise. 'How our grandmothers would have envied the carefree confidence with which modern women live every day to the full', one observes as she receives a drink from a young man, carefree in her very short playsuit and very high heels, with a Dutch-hat shielding her head from the sun.[49] The Kotex woman is also an accomplished tennis player, backhand at the ready, legs apart, 'with thousands of eyes watching every movement she is confident, comfortable and carefree'.[50] However, change was on the way and in 1942 the Kotex woman had begun to represent the working-class ignored by Modess. She is operating a machine, and finding 'comfort is half the battle. As you take up action stations Kotex contributes perfection in comfort'.[51] This Kotex woman represents the hundreds who released men from the factories for war combat by joining one of the many

---

46   'To meet the requirements of the modern woman', *The Brisbane Courier*, 15 March 1932, p. 18 and 26 April 1932, p. 15.
47   'At such times take care', 'Woman's Realm', supplement to *The Mercury*, 21 April 1937, p. 10s.
48   'The poise of confidence', 'Woman's Magazine' supplement to *The Argus*, 8 February 1941, p. 9s.
49   'Carefree confidence', 'Woman's Magazine' supplement to *The Argus*, 12 April 1941, p. 9s.
50   'Spotlight confidence' 'Woman's Magazine' supplement to *The Argus*, 13 September 1941, p. 9s.
51   'Comfort is half the battle', 'Woman's Magazine', supplement to *The Argus*, 21 March 1942, p. 5s.

auxiliary services such as munitions manufacture.[52] The theme is repeated with the Kotex woman, in uniform, cleaning the bonnet of an official-looking vehicle.[53]

The effects of the war on raw material imports were noticeable from mid-1942. Johnson and Johnson curtailed the activities of the Modess woman and a simple notice headed 'Modess shortage' explains why:

> The present shortage of Modess sanitary napkins is not as generally believed the result of undue rationing of imports by the Australian Govt. The cause, chiefly, is lack of shipping space. Raw materials for sanitary napkins naturally get left behind when war goods compete with them for space in ships coming to Australia. Supplies of Modess will be low for a few more weeks, after which larger quantities are confidently expected to be available.[54]

Johnson and Johnson were to be disappointed. The notice was repeated in August, and again in November, this time appearing in the main body of *The Mercury* rather than in the women's supplement, reiterating that supplies still remained on overseas docks awaiting space on Australian-bound ships and that the shortage would continue.[55] However, three weeks later the Modess woman returned, working as a nurse in a distinctly American uniform, but not tending war casualties. Rather, she is dramatically masked to weigh a baby, commenting that 'a nurse has to be on her toes in the baby ward! That's why on "difficult days" I'm doubly grateful to Miracle Modess. It has a wonderfully soft filler of fluff'. It is difficult to know if the supplies had arrived, or a desperate substitute 'fluff' had been created, in the manner of Kimberly-Clark's First World War Cellucotton, to provide Johnson and Johnson with their 'Miracle'.[56] As Christmas 1942 approached, advertising shifted to memories of past leisure with the Modess woman smilingly reclining on a chaise longue, her legs covered by a full-length satin evening skirt, her arms raised to support a cushion behind her head, sighing 'comfort, it's wonderful ...

52   Marilyn Lake, 'Freedom, fear and the family', in Patricia Grimshaw, Marilyn Lake, Ann McGrath, Marian Quartly, *Creating a Nation*, McPhee Gribble Publishers, Penguin Books, Ringwood, 1994, pp. 256–7, 259.
53   'Comfort is half the battle', *The Argus*, 2 May 1942, p. 5.
54   'Modess shortage', *The Mercury*, 22 July 1942, p. 6.
55   'Modess shortage', *The Mercury* 12 August 1942, p. 8; 'Supplies still limited', *The Mercury*, 13 November 1942, p. 6.
56   'Try it now', *The Mercury*, 27 November 1942, p. 7.

particularly on "difficult days".[57] The representation of the leisured woman in wartime may have had some association with the 1942–1943 influx of many thousand American servicemen to Australia, which the historian Marilyn Lake argues offered young women the opportunity for sexual romance, their particular danger zone during the war years.[58] The following year, 1943, reflected more focus on wartime Australia with the young Kotex woman seen initially holding a spanner, hands on hips. Her appearance coincides with the introduction of industrial conscription for Australian women who were either single or divorced. It was also a time of increased feminist activity with the goal of advancing women toward greater participation in public life. Readers are informed that 'women enlisted in the fighting services must have the comfort and security of Kotex for maximum efficiency. We are sorry that it is impossible to fully supply civilian needs as well but we trust the day is not far off when Kotex will be available for all of us'.[59] The young Kotex woman is later seen in two versions of auxiliary uniform: that of factory worker, and of the armed forces, captioned 'service is the theme today' signifying the service Kotex has given women in the Services, with reference to the absorbency advantages of Cellucotton.[60]

Kotex chose to continue an advertising presence but Johnson and Johnson's Modess woman was conspicuously absent from newspapers for the duration of the war. Kotex employed two strategies to identify as the 'tried, tested, and true' product – the one most in touch with women's changing lives – by using the young Kotex servicewoman in the present, and the other linking the product and women in the past. Readers were reminded of women's struggles to achieve freedom, socially and militarily, at the time of the Great War, when 'only daring women bobbed their hair' and 'women marched in suffrage parades'; and how lack of cotton for surgical dressings in army hospitals had led to the invention of Cellucotton surgical dressings, appropriated by nurses to use as sanitary pads, a story both celebrated and promoted as a freedom bestowed on women by Kotex.[61] The series continued, recollecting the fashion of the body-skimming skirts of the 1930s, their appearance concurrent with the introduction of Kotex'

---

57   'Comfort, it's wonderful', Woman's Realm supplement to *The Mercury*, 4 December 1942, p. 7s.
58   Lake in Grimshaw et al (1994), pp. 261–262.
59   'Priority for the women's services', *The Argus*, 18 January 1943, p. 6. See also Lake (1994), p. 260.
60   'Yesterday's fashions', *The Argus*, 13 May 1943, p. 6.
61   'Can you date this fashion?' *The Argus*, 2 March 1943.

'flat pressed ends' to facilitate concealment of the pad in situ, and the use of a 'Consumers' Testing Board' of 600 women in 1937, who approved the 'double duty safety centre ... developed to prevent roping and twisting' in Kotex pads.[62] These reminders of progress past were intended to placate women for the present problems of supply. Kotex would not relinquish the place it held in women's minds, although young girls' experiencing menarche would use the time-honoured menstrual cloth of washable towelling or similar fabric.

By 1944 there was a suggestion that women's optimism about the progress of the war had to be maintained, and Kotex constructed a tomorrow for their Woman, through futurist fashion, as the dream to off-set wartime rationing. Illustrations show her alone against the night sky and a sleek twin-level aircraft. She, and the reader, are asked, 'will an evening date see you stepping from a shining taxi of the skies ... your shoes glistening gold or metal, light and flexible as the air itself? Research by Kotex ... insures that you benefit from constant new developments'.[63] Next we see her, alone in her futuristic home, all her wartime experiences reduced to a 'model kitchen' in which she wears 'resilient cork-soled shoes', and 'heat resisting gloves', and the reminder that 'women never imagined they could be comfortable on difficult days. But Kotex changed all that'.[64]

Examples of increased independence by women, including attitudes toward their bodies, were further promoted through tampon advertisements. Johnson and Johnson used the teacher and the nurse as likely representatives of modern women who understand their physiology. The nurse comments that 'it would be silly for a nurse not to keep up with modern ideas' and that 'Modess had brought out Meds ... the best tampons I've ever used – and the only tampon in individual applicators ...'[65] The teacher, standing in front of a globe and holding a book, tells the reader that 'ancient history is my subject but not when it comes to sanitary protection. I'm all for the modern internal way'.[66] There were no notices published regarding shortage of supplies, but this would appear so because advertisements were suspended until 1946, and Tampax, imported from England, remained unavailable throughout the war years until 1947.[67]

---

62 'Can you date this fashion?' *The Argus*, 13 and 17 April 1943.
63 'Fashions of the future', *The Argus*, 13 March 1944, p. 6.
64 'Fashions of the future', *The Argus*, 11 May 1944, p. 8.
65 'Why I switched to Meds by a nurse', *The Argus*, 14 April 1943, p. 8.
66 'Why I switched to Meds by a school teacher', *The Argus*, 21 April 1943, p. 8.
67 'Tampax is back', 'Woman's magazine', supplement to *The Argus*, 9 February 1947, p. 20.

The post-war years were times of reconstruction culturally, socially and economically, with immigration programs attracting British families and major developmental projects progressing with a labour force significantly made up of non-British refugees and migrants from southern European countries, many of the women finding work in factories.[68] The war years for these women had meant far greater deprivation than a shortage of sanitary pads, but advertisements showed them vignettes of the life enjoyed by the Kotex woman: her femininity, her slinky long evening gowns, her stylish hair piled high, the text describing her as poised and self-assured, wanting the luxury that all women craved, and finding it in Kotex. The younger, carefree, Kotex girl played tennis, skied and leapt out of a canoe, watched admiringly by her boyfriend, and totally confident of 'no telltale outlines'.[69] The Modess woman continued to be constructed as leisured, sophisticated, elegantly groomed, always in the public space but never as a maternal figure. Her younger counterpart replicates the Kotex girl, also playing tennis. She is seen dressed in casual pants and top with hair in a pony-tail, or short-haired in checked capris, top and print scarf, espadrilles on feet. The Modess woman is 'modern', 'hard to please', 'confident' in her choice of 'softer, safer, economical' pads and the Modess girl is 'gay and carefree', 'smart', 'active', 'busy', and 'discriminating' in her choice of sanitary napkin.[70]

Tampons had a much greater advertising presence from 1947, the need for product promotion possibly reflecting prejudices found by historians Barbara Brookes and Margaret Tennant in their studies of New Zealand women, which indicated tampon use by virgins remained limited until the 1960s.[71] Once again two age groups of women were targeted. The 1946 Meds girl becomes the young mother, indicating social awareness by the

68   Lake in Grimshaw et al (1994), p. 272–273.

69   'Not a shadow of doubt', *Sydney Morning Herald* 25 October 1947, p. 12 and 11 November 1947, p. 13; 'Carefree', *Australian Women's Weekly,* 26 September 1951, p. 37; 26 March 1952, p. 10.

70   'Modern women prefer Modess', *The Argus,* 11 February 1948, p. 7; 'More and yet more women are changing', *The Argus* 30 May 1954, p. 22; 'Women who know are hard to please', *The Mercury,* 7 October 1950, p. 14; 'Each year more and more women look forward to Holiday Time', *The Mercury* 18 December 1954, p. 8; 'Just as important as the selection of a new season's gown', *The Mercury,* 29 October 1954; 'More Australian women buy Modess', *Sun-Herald* 29 November 1953, p. 52; 'Gay and carefree is the modern miss', 'Woman's Magazine' supplement to *The Argus,* 21 December 1948, p. 6s; 'Comfort's the keynote', *The Mercury,* 5 April 1952.

71   Barbara Brookes and Margaret Tennant, 'Making girls modern: Pakeha women and menstruation in New Zealand, 1930–70, *Women's History review,* vol. 7, no. 4, 1998, pp. 575–576.

manufacturers and caution in promoting the product to virgins.[72] In one advertisement an older woman is seen handing an apple to a glamorous younger one, captioned 'Go merrier with Meds'. Alongside is a smaller sketch of a young girl walking her dog and the text continues, 'women who long to try new fashioned protection will find the "small diameter" Meds Slender the perfect way to begin'. Clearly Johnson and Johnson were seeking ways to reach young, unmarried consumers.[73] They continued a series showing women encouraging each other to try Meds, the activities of these women illustrating a growing independence and awareness. Women are mobile, driving cars that may be their own – 'you can go anywhere, anytime, with Meds'.[74] They play tennis and golf, they push heavily laden wheelbarrows with 'the accent on freedom' and are informed of 'comfort and economy', 'protection and extra safety' and 'safety and economy', reassuring women who still remained uncertain about tampon use.[75]

By 1952 Johnson and Johnson began to openly contest the widely held social belief that tampons destroyed virginity, omitting reference to safety and replacing it with 'enlightenment'. The Meds girl wears a modest one-piece swimsuit under a cover-up: 'Single girls? Certainly. Medical evidence shows that any normal full-grown girl can wear Meds'. Moreover '4 out of 5 doctors report it is safe to swim on "those days" provided the water is not cold'.[76]

The change of promotional strategy is evidence of wider social change in thought about the young female body. In comparison, Tampax used the word 'safety' less in promotional texts, ensuring that 'freedom' became synonymous with their tampon. The Tampax woman of 1947 and 1948 has 'true loveliness' springing 'from confidence, from assurance, from the knowledge of freedom'. She plays active sport, and strides out in winter, hands in pockets and bag over shoulder, or is dressed more formally in a city, exuding independence and confidence. Apart from male-partnered social dancing, she is alone, and outside the domestic environment, reflecting the independence and individuality the war years gave to Australian women.[77]

---

72 'Free as the wind', *The Mercury*, 20 November 1946, p. 10.
73 'Go anywhere', 'Woman's Magazine', supplement to *The Argus*, 19 October 1948, p. 6s.
74 'You can go anywhere', *The Mercury*, 22 May 1946, p. 3.
75 'Accent on freedom', *The Mercury*, 27 February 1946, p. 5; 'Accent on Freedom', *The Argus*, 25 May 1946, p. 22 and 20 December 1947, p. 10.
76 'The beach? Why yes! Any day for me', *The Australian Women's Weekly*, 26 March 1952, p. 47.
77 'To women who love freedom', 'Woman's Magazine', supplement to *The Argus*, 12 March 1947, p. 21; 'Make a date with freedom', 'Woman's Magazine', supplement to *The Argus*,

For nearly 30 years the sanitary hygiene companies constructed women characterised by an absence of domestic environment, the two exceptions being the futuristic kitchen at the end of the war, when housing was desperately short,[78] and the mother–daughter series for *Marjorie May's Twelfth Birthday*. Consequently, the loudest message for young adolescents looking at the advertisements, regardless of their ability to read or speak English, was that women who had wealth and lived enviable lives used these products. However, there were two other significant messages. One, that menarche and menstruation did not interrupt normal activities and, two, that concealment was mandatory. So the recurring terms 'security, safety, confidence, protection' signify menstruation to be 'other' to normality, which is characterised by the state of non-bleeding.

Immigrant women brought their cultural beliefs about the female body, often contesting knowledge transmitted by welfare bodies and sanitary product manufactures. For instance, Rosalia's ignorance at menarche was common to Italian immigrants, as Brumberg noted with older Italian-Americans. Their cultural beliefs determined continuing use of washable menstrual cloths because disposable absorbents were thought to hamper the good flow that indicated health and potential fertility.[79] Qing, in Hong Kong, recalled that her mother, a midwife, never spoke of menstruation, and the sociologist Cordia Ming-Yeuk Chu explains the reason. Chinese culture regards both menstruation and sexual activity as being unclean, consequently the transition of girl to woman by menarche signals her role as potential sex partner. Social rules governing women's behaviour include avoidance of reference to any unclean state, a custom giving rise to unease between mothers and daughters.[80] Lack of maternal explanation about menarche and menstruation can also cause resentment, as Wani in Indonesia remembered feeling, but psychologist Deanna Dorman Logan's study of the menarcheal experience in the 1970s indicates that Indonesian girls, informed about menstruation by their mothers, reported a need for greater biological and practical explanation of the whole subject, a desire echoed in the study by

---

16 April 1947, p. 14; 'To women of action who love freedom', 'Woman's Magazine', supplement to *The Argus*, 17 September 1947, p. 18; 'Beauty is not looks alone', 'Woman's Magazine', supplement to *The Argus*, 1 June 1948, p. 6; 'Beauty has a better chance today', 'Woman's Magazine', supplement to *The Argus*, 10 August 1948, p. 6.

78   Lake in Grimshaw et al (1994), p. 274.

79   Brumberg (1993), p. 120–121.

80   Cordia Ming-Yeuk Chu, 'Menstrual beliefs and practices of Chinese women', *Journal of the Folklore Institute*, vol. 17, no. 1, 1980, p. 50.

psychologist Ayse K. Askul on the menarcheal experience of women from diverse cultures.[81]

Conclusion

The desire of pubescent girls for accurate knowledge about menarche and menstruation was widespread but the manner in which this information was obtained depended on cultural factors. Interviews demonstrate that between the 1930s and 1960s, the transmission was oral, controlled by women – mothers, friends, older sisters or cousins – and combined personal or anecdotal experience with traditional lore. By comparison, in Australia until the 1940s, many mothers shared a commonality with mothers in other cultures in the suppression of pre-menarcheal information. This was challenged by the publication of informative booklets, although maternal control continued to be held over daughters' access to the publications. The content of early menstrual education texts, including the non-commercial Father and Son Welfare Movement 1932–1949, reflected both religious and medical influence, but as sanitary hygiene companies developed further texts they incorporated the influence of US 'teen culture', with an increasing emphasis on the menstruant being sexually attractive, an aspect of maturation remembered by interviewees as causing considerable maternal concern in cultures that value virginity until marriage.

Interviews made evident the role of peer-group friends as menstrual informants. Their experience-based knowledge contributed to the attitudes formed toward menarche and menstruation by interviewees, a knowledge obviously valued by many women. However, the Australian-edition text *Marjorie May's Twelfth Birthday* makes clear that girls in the 1930s and 1940s were not encouraged to share their menstrual experience. Later texts, both booklet and advertising, acknowledged that it was part of pubescent life.

Learning by observing a menstruating older sister was recalled by interviewees as a lesson in the normality of menstruation. This was almost certainly a part of the Australian girls' menstrual education too, but less effective as the use of shared bedrooms decreased, menstrual absorbents improved, and washing machines became part of domestic life. Consequently, observation shifted from the actual to the fictional, through magazine

---

81   Deana Dorman Logan, 'The menarche experience in twenty-three foreign countries', *Adolescence*, vol. 15, no. 58, 1980, p. 251. See also Ayse K. Uskal, 'Women's menarche stories from a multicultural sample', *Social Science and Medicine*, vol. 59, no. 4, 2004, p. 674.

advertisements promoting sanitary hygiene products which constructed menstruating young women according to the wider social context, but always as capable, glamorous, and middle-class Anglo-Australians, engaged in a series of enviable activities, their menstrual lives enhanced by pads and tampons. Language used in accompanying information was sanitised to conceal the reality of periods at a time when young women were being encouraged to break free from the persisting 19th-century illness construction, and participate in the exciting moment of menarche and normal, healthy, active, menstrual life.

The waves of immigration that brought multicultural interviewees to Australia also brought old traditions associated with menarche and menstruation. Their daughters, experiencing menarche in their new country did so according to maternal cultural beliefs, with none of the menstrual educational texts discussed providing any other than an Anglo-English perspective. Had the cultural traditions of the major immigrant groups toward menarche and menstruation been acknowledged, and briefly explained, both Anglo-Australian and immigrant girls would have been helped to bridge cultural differences through understanding the non-biological meanings attributed to this phenomenon.

Chapter 8

FROM MENARCHE TO WHERE?

Now it's a different story.[1]

Inevitably women's memories of menarche and the diverse cultural meanings attributed to it prompted me to think of the future and what this first menstrual period might mean for young girls in coming years. It is highly unlikely that the implications of menarche will carry the same significance as it did for my interviewees, whose menarcheal experience occurred in the 1930s–1960s, but where the changes in thought and attitude toward the menstrual process will be focused remains uncertain. Although regional and cultural differences are significant when considering such a future, it is the impact of media technology over the past two decades that is influencing rapid social change and the sharing of previously private knowledge and thoughts about the menstrual process, although in an uneven way according to accessibility. So while evidence indicates that women in the West are increasingly choosing to practise some form of menstrual suppression[2] it is not yet clear whether the millions of women in developing countries, who still live menstrual lives in circumstances of extreme hardship, might accept such an option.

---

1   Alisha, c.14 years old at menarche, India c.1943.
2   Jennifer Gorman Rose, Joan C. Chrisler, and Samantha Couture, 'Young women's attitudes toward continuous use of oral contraceptives: the effect of priming positive attitudes toward menstruation on women's willingness to suppress menstruation', *Health Care for Women International*, vol. 29, no. 7, 2008 and Christine M. Read, 'New regimes with combined oral contraceptive pills – moving away from traditional 21/7 cycles', *The European Journal of Contraception and Reproductive Health Care*, vol. 15, no. 2, 2010, and Alecia J. Grieg, Michelle A. Palmer, Lynne M. Chepulis, 'Hormonal contraceptive practices in young Australian women (<25 years) and their possible impact on menstrual frequency and iron requirements', *Sexual and Reproductive Healthcare*, vol. 1, no. 3, 2010. See also Shelley Gare, 'Secret women's business', *The Age Good Weekend*, 1 May 2010, p. 51. Gare reports on interviews with Dr Terri Foran, medical director of Family Planning, NSW, and Dr Elizabeth Farrell, Jean Hailes Foundation for Women's Health, Melbourne.

While it is apparent, among the changes affecting girls, that new concepts of menstrual management are creating conditions for further evolution of menstrual practices, progress comes at a cultural cost. For instance, successfully teaching menstrual management breaks down the cultural tradition of silence surrounding menstruation, allowing women a voice in community decision-making in matters relating to menarche and menstruation – a small start to wider participation. In other respects there is a certain resonance with the changes affecting young Western women from the early 20th century. The difference today is the social context in which these events are occurring in developing countries, including the influential reach of Western media as a learning device and a growing awareness of the harmful effects of the ever-increasing quantity of disposable menstrual absorbents on the environment.

In the preceding chapters I have examined the layers of meaning attributed to menarche and menstruation within various cultures. I have shown how medical thought in ancient societies constructed menarche as the symbol of instability in transition from child to reproductive woman, and how its onset was thought to be fraught with danger, particularly if any deviation from the culturally established norm occurred. Having defined normality, medical treatment of any deviation was instituted and surviving documentation provides evidence that menarche, specifically among the wealthier strata of societies, has a long history of being considered a medical concern. In the late 19th century medical debate over the effect of education on the future reproductive capabilities of middle-class young women included the voice of a woman medical practitioner who refuted the assertions made by her male counterparts. At the same time the rise of the hygiene movement and the development of disposable absorbents, initially marketed as surgical dressings and medical accessories for accouchement, became recognised by manufacturers as having the growth potential of a sanitary hygiene industry. Product promotion diversified to education, under medical supervision, introducing girls to a menstrual practice based on concealment of the biological process.

Until the Second World War, changes in menstrual thought and practice mainly affected girls and young women in wealthier urban areas, many of whom would, or already had, moved from the domestic sphere to the public workplace. Their menstrual management was, in part, facilitated by urban infrastructure in large towns and cities where running water and flushing toilets had been the norm for over a century. Household waste was regularly collected by city or town council employees and concerns about environmental degradation remained in the future. For the most part, however, girls living in less developed rural areas of Western countries continued to be influenced by older traditions, including belief in the dichotomous power of menarcheal blood to either cause harm or create vulnerability to harm. In some cultures, and in some religious belief systems, these beliefs are still transmitted inter-generationally at the time of menarche and are the cause for ritualistic seclusion and the symbolism of ceremony. Nor has this menstrual lore been entirely ignored by Western scientists, who sought a pharmacological basis for the belief that harm was caused to certain plants by the menstrual touch.

Where a culture entrenches certain practices, social change and the acceptance of scientific and technological advancements influencing such change, does not occur evenly or in isolation but within varying contexts of national economic systems and political and social power. The prospective financial gain by interested individuals and corporations, the recognition and reward of researchers, and the seemingly unequal relations between the testers and the tested at the level of trials to determine efficacy and potential development of the new, are also issues in any future outcomes for women in developing countries. Thus, while it is possible that menarche may continue being a cause of ritual seclusion for some, or celebration for others, it will depend on the continued relevance of existing cultural and religious belief systems or on the proliferation of fundamentalism. Alternatively, following the patterns of change in developed countries, menarche may become an increasingly isolated event, serving only to signify biological maturation, perhaps without further menstruation, or with controlled menstruation, as is beginning to be practised in Western countries. This latter movement is the result of advancements in biological research over the past 60 years, which have revolutionised Western women's lives, and continue to do so, and will probably become an even larger part of the lives of young women in developing nations.

Today, poorer women in developing countries are being educated in hygienic menstrual practice for reasons of health. This is one of the current changes occurring at a community level that can be strongly resisted at the cultural level. For example, in 2008 the British Medical Journal reported the deaths of two young women in rural Nepal during menstrual seclusion. The deaths were attributed to extremes of weather and pre-existing colds and diarrhoea which worsened fatally during their four or five days in an outdoor shed lacking any facilities. This situation was common enough to have had a decision made by the Supreme Court of Nepal in 2005 declaring menstrual seclusion, or *chhaupadi*, illegal.[3] The response in 2008–2009 was a study carried out in four urban and rural districts of Nepal, which sought to identify problems associated with menstruation in 204 post-menarcheal adolescent schoolgirls.[4] Three major areas of concern were identified. First, the cultural influences affecting knowledge and beliefs, including the silence surrounding menstruation and the shock of menarche. This particularly affects girls belonging to the caste groups *Bahun*, *Chhetri* and *Newar*, who are ritually secluded in the dark at menarche for 7 to 11 days, during which they may not see either the sun or male relatives. For other girls the polluting power of menarche and menstruation is most commonly expressed in exclusion from religious activities and prohibition of food preparation. Yet there is some evidence that young girls are questioning cultural beliefs, with one relating that when menstruating and unobserved she touches all that is prohibited to her, with no repercussion beyond her own scepticism.[5] The second concern is the way in which girls construct menstruation as an abnormal, often painful, physical condition causing them stress from fear of staining at school, and through absenteeism, with one girl from Lalitpur in Nepal, caught in the conflict between managing her period and performing well in her class IX exams, commenting that she wishes she did not have to menstruate, but she 'knows' that is impossible.[6] A major issue is the link between menstrual hygiene practice and school absenteeism, attributed to lack of affordable sanitary pads, water and proper washing facilities for girls, who need privacy to wash both body and menstrual cloth after walking long distances to school. The other serious lack is an effective disposal system, resulting in used menstrual absorbents being discarded in the toilet pan, with resultant blockage or, in rural areas, being thrown into streams, with subsequent environmental implications.[7]

The Nepal example can be translated to other non-industrialised societies. There are many African and south Asian countries that have largely ignored

---

3   Khagendra Dahal, 'Nepalese woman dies after banishment to shed during menstruation', 'News' in *British Medical Journal*, vol. 337, 22 November 2008, p. 1194.
4   Om Gautam, 'Is menstrual hygiene and management an issue for adolescent school girls in Nepal?', *Regional Conference on Appropriate Water Supply, Sanitation and Hygiene (WASH) Solutions for Informal Settlements and Marginalised Communities, Katmandu, Nepal, 19–21 May 2010*, p. 170. Gautam is a social development adviser to WaterAid, Nepal. http://www.nec.edu.np/delphe/pdf/conference1pdf#page=192
5   Gautam (2010), pp. 175, 178–179.
6   Gautam (2010), p, 180.
7   Gautam, pp. 181–183.

the need women have for facilities for menstrual hygiene, partly as a result of the cultural silence around the subject of menstruation. In India, UNICEF[8] has taken steps to break the silence about menstruation and to teach girls and women about menstrual hygiene in a shared association with the Government of India's Total Sanitation Campaign and other similar programs. The result is a small booklet intended for girls and their families, titled *Sharing Simple Facts*, published in 2008 with translations into Hindi and other Indian languages planned. The booklet explains the physiological and emotional aspects of puberty, arguing against cultural belief that menstrual blood is impure, and integrating references to traditional menstrual practices that are unnecessary and undesirable in today's communities. Menstruating girls are encouraged to participate in normal school activities and to negotiate at home over practices such as segregation of the sexes. Modernity is the weapon of persuasion and girls might point out that change is happening in households where parents are educated and progressive in outlook. Menarche ceremonies are fewer, attributed to the embarrassment caused to a modern young girl through advertising her newly arrived fertility, but also because of the health risks of early marriage and childbirth. Once again, modernity has influenced a lessening of the practice of menstrual seclusion, explained as a rest time from chores but now difficult to observe in nuclear families. Commercially manufactured sanitary hygiene products, familiar in the West, are listed together with those made by Self Help Groups (SHG), but there is no mention of tampons, which are culturally inappropriate for virgin girls. A comprehensive description of correct sanitary absorbent disposal methods is provided, with the warning that menstrual pads pollute the environment and generate problems for solid waste management.[9] *Sharing Simple Facts* reflects Western input in the text, suggesting menstrual traditions are disappearing, but it has been pointed out that although schooling may provide a sense of choice for young girls, cultural traditions still obstruct change and explain school absence during menstruation, particularly among South- East Asian Hindus. Even now, in south India, menarche signals the end of schooling for many Hindu girls because marriage is arranged at, or soon after, the first period. Tradition also dictates that Hindu girls will avoid washing facilities at schools because of the risk of menstrual

---

8   United Nations International Children's Emergency Fund.
9   *Sharing Simple Facts: Useful Information about Menstrual Health and Hygiene*, UNICEF and Department of Drinking Water Supply, Ministry of Rural Development, New Delhi, 2008.

pollution to water sources, and those with access to flushing toilets will avoid them in case of blood staining.[10] In the rural Shimla district of India, a study among predominantly Christian school girls, age 9–15 years, by interns and medical practitioners in 1994–1995, indicates girls are using clean home-made menstrual cloths or commercially-made sanitary pads in place of unwashed menstrual cloths. Fewer girls are ignorant about menstruation, reflecting better communication on the subject between the generations, but few learn from teachers or from books. Possibly as a result of Christian influence, less than 25 per cent of girls follow traditional menstrual prohibitions relating to physical contact with others, food preparation and religious devotions.[11] In Mumbai, a study among rural women immigrants to the city, carried out from 1996 to 2000, reveals health problems due to crowded living conditions and lack of sanitary hygiene facilities. Women are prevented from washing their used menstrual cloths, which they bundle unwashed for re-use. In rural areas cloths are traditionally buried to prevent any practice of witchcraft but as urban slums lack burial space and privacy for such disposal, cloths are now thrown away. By necessity, changes to nuclear-family living conditions have also caused most of these women to discard the menstrual taboos of entering the kitchen and handling food.[12]

The habit of reusing menstrual cloths appears widespread and the reasons for the practice are similar. In Bangladesh the majority of women use pieces of old saris for menstrual cloths, washing them in a clay pot or basin of used water without soap, and hiding them to dry in a dark place, well away from the sight of men who might be harmed by them, according to cultural beliefs. The common practice of reusing damp menstrual cloths, resulting in vaginal and urinary tract infections, emphasises the need for girls and women to be educated in matters of menstrual hygiene.[13] Subsequently,

---

10 Thérèse Mahon and Maria Fernandes, 'Menstrual hygiene in South Asia: a neglected issue for WASH (water, sanitation and hygiene) programmes', *Gender and Development*, vol. 18, no. 1, 2010, pp. 103–104. Fernandes is Programme Officer, WaterAid, Regional India, Bhopal and Mahon is Asian Regional Programme Officer, WaterAid, for India, Nepal, Bangladesh and Pakistan.

11 A.K. Gupta, A. Vatsayan, S.K. Ahluwalia, R.K. Sood, S.R. Mazta, R. Sharma, 'Age at menarche, menstrual knowledge and practice in the apple belt of Shimla hills', *Journal of Obstetrics and Gynaecology*, vol. 16, no. 6, 1996, pp. 548–550.

12 Suneela Garg, Nandini Sharma, Ragini Sahay, 'Socio-cultural aspects of menstruation in an urban slum in Delhi, India', *Reproductive Health matters*, vol. 9, no. 17, 2001, pp. 16–17, 21–22. The authors are socio-epidemiologists.

13 Rokeya Ahmed and Kabita Yesmin, 'Menstrual hygiene: breaking the silence', in *WaterAid Beyond Construction: a Collection of Case Studies from Sanitation and Hygiene Promotion Practitioners in South Asia*, James Wicken, Joep Verhagen, Christine

in 2005, Sanitation, Hygiene Education and Water Supply in Bangladesh (SHEWAB) developed a strategy for educating girls and women in menstrual management. Initially, cultural silence toward menstruation prevented the necessary communication between men and women at training level, but the cultural embargo was solved by constructing an educational program in partnership with Non-Government Organisations (NGOs), including UNICEF. As a result, community workers of both genders are now trained to address menstrual hygiene management at village level.[14] The program, supported by local government and school management groups, centres on meetings attended by girls and women, including women teachers, held in local schools. The trained community workers provide menstrual hygiene education and support to the groups of women, inviting them to contribute ideas to planning water supplies and women-specific toilet facilities for their menstrual needs.[15] SHEWAB has trained community workers to teach the benefits of disposable menstrual pads but, as they remain widely unavailable, hygiene practices taught relate only to menstrual cloths.[16]

Social changes brought about by industrialisation have alienated many young girls from their families, and Members of the Alliance for African Women's Initiative in Ghana, (AFAWIGH), draw attention to several issues resulting from rapid urbanisation and widespread family dispersal. One problem discussed is young girls' ignorance about menstrual matters. Previously at menarche a girl was taught about her expected future behaviour by her mother and other women of her community. Her menarche ceremony, conducted by the 'queen mothers' of the community, entailed instruction about menstrual and sexual hygiene and marriage, but today's girls reach menarche earlier and without the social structures in place. They are left to make their own discoveries about their physical change. The women Members made the following recommendations. One, that programs be

---

Sijbesma, Carmen da Silva, Peter Ryan (eds), WaterAid London, 2008, pp. 283–284, http:// www.wateraid.org/documents/ch21_menstrual_hygiene_breaking_the_silence.pdf. See also Shaheen Akhter, 'Knowledge, attitudes and practices on reproductive health and rights of urban and rural women in Bangladesh', Yokohama National University Repository, 2007, pp. 138–139, http://www.kamome.lib.ynu. ac.jp/dspace/bitstream/10131/3157/1/3-131-akhter.pdf

14   Kathryn Seymour, 'Bangladesh: tackling menstrual hygiene taboos', Sanitation and Hygiene, Case Study 10, http://www.UNICEF.org/wash/files10_case_study_BANGLADESH_4web.pdf, 2008, pp. 1–2. The program is run by the Sanitation, Hygiene Education and Water Supply in Bangladesh(SHEWAB) backed by UNICEF. See also Ahmed and Yesmin (2008), pp. 284–285.

15   Ahmed and Yesmin (2008), pp. 285–286.

16   Seymour (2008), pp. 1–4.

introduced to teach pre-pubescent primary school girls about menstruation and menstrual hygiene management and be followed through at secondary school as part of adolescent and reproductive health. Two, that calls be made for attitudinal change in religious organisations that prohibit menstruating girls from participating in prayers and religious activities because of the negative effects on the girls. Three, that calls be made for public education to reduce negative ideas surrounding menstruation, stemming from traditional beliefs and practices. Additional recommendations replicate those made in Bangladesh regarding the construction of girl-specific washing facilities at schools, with provision for disposal of menstrual pads. It is noted that girls' menstrual absorbents in Ghana include vegetable matter such as leaves, toilet paper, or bits of sacking, and that their knowledge of the hygienic advantages of disposable sanitary pads remains limited due to either poverty or unavailability.[17]

The situation in Ghana is echoed in Uganda with the NGO Forum for African Women Educationalists (FAWE) campaigning to break the prohibition on speaking about matters related to menstruation, and advocating cheaper sanitary absorbents to be sold at local markets. Menstrual hygiene problems are stated to be the largest single cause for girls dropping out of school and are attributed to lack of access to menstrual absorbents due to poverty and sustained cultural beliefs and attitudes.[18] Following a study made with 500 post-menarcheal girls in south-eastern Nigeria, recommendations include the use of the media in menstrual hygiene education. Also recommended is the promotion of menstrual education by women's associations and NGOs through women's conferences and seminars, and their assistance in the provision and distribution of pads at subsidised rates. Once again a call is made for the instruction of pre-menarcheal girls as part of the school curriculum, and for the provision of disposal facilities for used menstrual absorbents to combat menstrual absenteeism.[19]

---

17 'Sexual maturation and menstrual management practices associated with schoolgirls in Ghana', Alliance for African Women's Initiative, Ghana 2010, pp. 1–2, 4–5, http://afawigh.org/publication/sexual-maturation-and-menstrual-management-practices-associated-with-school-girls-in-ghana.html

18 Sowmyaa Bharadwaj and Archana Patkar, 'Menstrual hygiene and management in developing countries: taking stock', Junction Social, Mumbai, 2004, p. 11, http://www.mum.org/menhydev.htm

19 Uzochukwu Uzoma Aniebue, Patricia Nonelum Aniebue, Theophilus Ogochukwu Nwankwo, 'The impact of pre-menarcheal training on menstrual practices and hygiene of Nigerian schoolgirls', Pan African Medical Journal, vol. 1, no. 2, 2009, pp. 2–8, http:// www.panafrican-med-journal.com/content/article/2/9/full

The principal cause of girls dropping out of school in developing countries is indisputably linked to cultural beliefs and attitudes, but it is also one
of logistics caused by the problem of disposal of menstrual waste in areas of
extreme poverty. It is a widespread situation throughout the south Asian
area, including East Timor where an Australian Volunteers International
community worker, Sarah Angus, spoke of her proudest achievement being
the construction of a school toilet block in Uai-Bua because until then
menstruating girls would not attend school.[20] There is little doubt that the
betterment of women's lives and health begins at menarche, when good
menstrual hygiene practices, as well as an understanding of the body, can
be taught by trained instructors at community level. The system appears
effective but there is another aspect that has come under scrutiny. Financial
support for menstrual health campaigns has been given by various NGOs
and other corporations, including a guaranteed US$5 million by the
sanitary hygiene company Proctor and Gamble for menstrual education
and distribution of pads. The Clinton Global Initiative subsidises African
businesses with US$2.8 million to provide inexpensive pads to help girls
stay at school. The costs and benefits of these programs drew the attention of
economists Emily Oster and Rebecca Thornton, who argue that menstrual
hygiene products make little difference to girls' school attendance. They base
their assertion on two issues: that the reports of menstrual absenteeism from
school are anecdotal and lack hard evidence, and that a trial they ran in
the Chitwan area of Nepal with 198 participants provided evidence to the
contrary. Oster and Thornton contend their findings are due to their analysis
of the patterns of menstrual absence which fail to indicate any significant
impact on schooling, although it is noted that in the previous year 48.3 per
cent of the girls participating in the study reported menstrual absence due to
cramps, and 20 per cent remained at home because of concerns of mobility
and lack of washing facilities at school for washing menstrual rags.[21]

An additional randomised test against the known reasons for menstrual
absence from school, carried out by Oster and Thornton, studied the
efficacy of an advanced sanitary hygiene device known as the menstrual
cup. The cup, which collects menstrual blood rather than absorbing it, is
made from industrially manufactured silicone, bell-shaped, long-lasting,
washable, and reusable. It is inserted into the vagina without risk of toxic

---

20   Carolyn Webb, 'Christmas spirit knows no borders', *The Age*, 23 December 2010.
21   Emily Oster and Rebecca Thornton, 'Menstrual sanitary protection and school
      attendance: evidence from a randomized evaluation', *American Economic Journal:
      Applied Economics*, vol. 3, no. 1, 2011, pp. 91–92, 97–98.

shock.[22] Its use is evaluated in regard to school attendance with 100 girls taking part, of whom 50 were given a cup. The results show no change to the existing minimal school absence of 0.4 school days in the 180-day school year due to menstruation, but there is marked enthusiasm reported by the participants about their experience of the menstrual cup, its facilitation of mobility, and the time saved in washing and drying menstrual cloths. No reference is made to cultural views on virginity regarding the use of a vaginal device, nor is the number of Hindu participants known, although one mother–daughter decided not to accept the cup. Neither is there any way of proving the device was actually used.[23] However, the most concerning problem with Oster and Thornton's findings, which they argue may be generalised outside Nepal, is the risk of withdrawal of program funding, and the possible ripple effect on other projects related to good menstrual management for future health.

The issues of cultural acceptance, cost, accessibility and supervision are influential in acceptance of innovations such as the menstrual cup, which may alter the perceptions of girls and women to menstruation. These factors have yet to be studied. Meanwhile information about cultural menstrual practices continues to be collected, particularly by volunteer workers at times of social dislocation, providing information for immediate help and for shaping future policy. One example is Pakistan, following the earthquake in 2005, when thousands of Muslim women and girls in the tented villages were visited by Oxfam partner staff, proficient in the local language, to discuss their needs including those related to menstrual hygiene practice. The significance of the key issues identified is their relevance to all Muslim women in developing countries, including the absolute necessity for menstrual hygiene educators and sanitary engineers to be women. Additionally, community workers must understand the cultural attitudes dictating the silence surrounding menstruation, and the need for any discussions to be totally private and restricted to girls and women. Effective menstrual hygiene practice has to acknowledge the pollutant aspect of menstruation by requiring concealed disposal facilities for used sanitary pads to avoid public display. Menstrual cloths must be of dark fabric to conceal blood and washing facilities must be plumbed to conceal blood-stained water drainage.[24]

---

22 The menstrual cup used was manufactured by Mooncup and the authors do not declare receiving any financial support from them. See http://www.mooncup.co.uk
23 Oster and Thornton (2011), pp. 93, 94 and f.n 5, 95, 97, 99.
24 Jamila Nawaz, Shamma Lal, Saira Raza and Sarah House, 'Oxfam experience of providing screened toilet, bathing and menstruation units in its earthquake response in Pakistan', *Gender and Development*, vol. 18, no. 1, 2010, pp. 81–84.

This overview of the situation shows that many women in developing countries share poor menstrual practice for identical reasons based on cultural and religious traditions, including silence in matters of menstruation. There is evidence of the problem being managed in almost identical ways, through opening channels of communication within communities to provide girls with the knowledge of menarche, menstruation and good menstrual hygiene practice. Village women are becoming involved in planning facilities for women's menstrual needs, and being made aware of the availability and disposal of menstrual absorbents. Additionally, there is evidence that women working through NGO groups and women's associations are driving change in the developing south Asian and African countries referred to, as well as indications that young girls are questioning cultural traditions such as menstrual prohibition. Change caused by industrialisation and rural migration to overcrowded urban space has resulted in hardship for women trying to maintain cultural practices associated with menstruation, some of which have been discarded in new forms of nuclear family life.

Historian Andrew Shail argues the consciousness of late capitalism shapes ideas of waste in the minds of consumers, with disposable menstrual absorbents being the classic example of unending waste and equally unending manufacture, maintaining the system.[25] This is apparent in the growing demand for disposable menstrual absorbents among impoverished women in Bangladesh and the response in 1999 by the Bangladesh Rural Advancement Committee (BRAC). A manufacturing industry making disposable menstrual pads was established, offering paid women employees incentives for promotion and sales. The total daily output is 6,000 packets, each containing 12 looped pads of cotton-filled gauze, sterilised, and sealed in plastic packets. Sales are mainly to district health workers who on-sell door-to-door at a profit, but pads are also sold through local markets at greater profit, while undercutting known brands. Yet the problem of disposal remains unsolved. Used pads are thrown into a pit and covered with soil.[26] Similar enterprises have been developed in other areas, including in the Indian state of Chhattisgarh, where rural women in 50 villages have learned how to manufacture disposable cloth pads, which are discarded in a sanitary pit after use.[27]

---

25 Andrew Shail, '"Athough a woman's article": menstruant economics and creative waste', *Body and Society*, vol. 13, no. 4, 2007, pp. 86–87.
26 Bharadwaj and Patkar (2004), pp. 12–13. See also 'BRAC sanitary napkins and birthing kits', http://www.brac.net/content/social-enterprises-health
27 Mahon and Fernandes (2010), pp. 109–110.

Having made affordable disposable menstrual pads for poorer girls and women, and having informed millions about the association between menstrual hygiene practices and health, the issue of environmental awareness has emerged as a shared concern, not confined to developing countries but reaching into the minds of Australian and New Zealand women through conservational promotion and awareness-raising events. In the Melbourne suburb of Moreland, for example, Zero Waste for a Week Challenge was held in November 2010, during which time women in the community were made conscious of the annual landfill containing over 700 million tampons and 1 billion menstrual pads, together with their plastic packaging. Women were asked to consider reusable menstrual pads or menstrual cups in preference to disposable menstrual absorbents.[28] In New Zealand, Pip Lynch draws attention to a growing awareness of environmental degradation in alpine, bush and coastal terrain through the effects of disposable menstrual absorbents. Many of the manufactured products contain chlorine-bleached fluff-making kraft or sulphate pulp, with anti-bacterial properties capable of destroying healthy micro-flora in soil so that decomposition of buried pads and tampons is delayed, with potential effects on groundwater, vermin and flies. In addition, toxic chemicals released by synthetic products during degradation and incineration have the potential to cause toxic pollution. Women are recommended to consider alternative menstrual management, including use of the environmentally sound menstrual cup which has no harmful components.[29]

Education leading to change in menstrual management practice and avoidance of ecological degradation presents women in both developed and non-developed countries with challenges for the future. It might be argued that no menstrual absorbent, be it disposable or washable, is without hazard to health or environment. Furthermore women's menstrual life is longer. In 1976 R. V. Short drew attention to the earlier menarche and subsequent fertility experienced by girls in developed countries and how the socially imposed period of infertility, helped by contraception, allows intellectual maturity to catch up with that of the physical.[30] Girls in developing countries

---

28 Moreland City Council, 'Zero Waste for a Week Challenge' November 2010, www.more land.vic.gov.au/environment-and-waste/rubbish-collection/zero-waste-challenge.html
29 Pip Lynch, 'Menstrual waste in the backcountry', *Science for Conservation:35*, Department of Conservation, Wellington, 1996, pp. 5, 10–13.
30 R. V. Short, 'The evolution of human reproduction', *A Discussion on Contraceptives of the Future,* Royal Society, London, 1976, p. 11. Short is a Fellow of both the Royal College of Veterinary Surgeons and the Royal College of Gynaecologists. He

experience a later menarche, attributed to reduced body mass and its effect as an ovulation suppressant, the body's own contraceptive, not dissimilar to the effects of weight loss in anorexia nervosa-affected young women in Western nations.[31] As living conditions undergo change in developing countries, the future patterns of fertility may follow those of today's Western women with earlier menarche, reduced reproduction and lactation time, and an extended menstrual life of about 30 years. Most significantly, according to Short, this situation has neither evolutionary precedence nor genetic adaptation. Consequently it is in the interest of women's health to reduce bleeding. While this may be of limited impact in developed countries it could have considerable advantage for women in developing nations where protein deprivation and vulnerability to diseases such as malaria or hookworm reduces their potential for good health.[32]

Menstrual suppression was always possible with the 'Pill' from its initial government approval in 1957 as treatment for menstrual irregularities and infertility.[33] However, in the days before pregnancy kits were easily obtained from supermarkets, researcher and inventor Gregory Pincus and co-inventor gynaecologist John Rock believed that women would want a pseudo-period to reassure them they were not pregnant. Rock, a devout Catholic, wanted the Pill to duplicate the natural female bodily function, signifying it as a 'natural' combination of hormones that extended the theologically acceptable 'safe period' of a woman's reproductive cycle, of importance to Roman Catholic theologians who were opposed to artificial forms of fertility control.[34] So alternative dosage regimes of the drug to suppress menstruation

---

was Foundation Director of the Medical Research Council's Unit of Reproductive Biology in Edinburgh 1972–1982 and held the Chair in Reproductive Biology at Monash University, Melbourne 1982–1995. See also Rachel Blumstein Posner, 'Early menarche: a review of research on trends in timing, racial differences, etiology and psychosocial consequences', *Sex Roles,* vol. 54, nos 5–6, 2006, pp. 316, 320, which argues that social fear of emergent female sexuality led to G. Stanley Hall (1904) constructing the concept of the adolescent as a potential problem requiring behavioural therapy. Posner, a psychologist, contends the mean age of menarche in the US has been demonstrated to be unchanged over the past 50 years.

31   Short (1976), p. 14.
32   Short (1996), pp. 18–19.
33   For a history of the 'Pill' see historians Suzanne White Junod and Lara Marks, 'Women's trials: the approval of the first oral contraceptive pill in the United States and Great Britain', *Journal of the History of Medicine and Allied Sciences,* vol. 57, no. 2, 2002 and Victor A. Drill, 'History of the first oral contraceptive', *Journal of Toxicology and Environmental Health,* Part A, vol. 3, no 1, 1977, pp. 133–134. Drill was Director of Biological Research 1953–1970 for G. D. Searle and Company, developers of the first oral contraceptive, Enovid, successfully trialled in 1956.
34   Malcolm Gladwell, 'John Rock's Error', *New Yorker Annals of Medicine,* 13 March 2000, pp. 53–55. See also David F. Archer, 'Menstrual-cycle related symptoms:

were not included in the information sheet enclosed in every packet of oral contraceptives sold. Furthermore, medical practitioners rarely explained to patients that if they wished to avoid a period they could ignore the differently coloured placebo (sugar) pills in the tablet pack. It was left to the agency of women to specifically ask their doctors for guidance pending particular activities – a honeymoon, a holiday, sports participation – and they would then be advised.[35] The withdrawal bleed for one week in every 28 days was considered by many women to be menstruation and the fact that there is little endometrial lining to shed continues to be poorly understood.[36]

Should women understand more about a drug that has such profound effect on their bodies? The idea of menstrual suppression creates considerable debate from health professionals, some funded by pharmaceutical companies, studying women's responses to the concept.[37] Common to their findings is a marked lack of knowledge about the menstrual process by young women, associated with a lack of understanding of how oral contraception suppresses bleeding. Many young women gain their knowledge of menstrual suppression from popular magazines and the media, with resultant biases reflective of marketing promotion.[38] Their shared concerns include side-effects and long-term effects on health and fertility, but some also fear menstrual suppression will prevent them recognising pregnancy.[39] For others, the influence of traditional ideas about menstruation being the vital essence of femininity,

a review of the rationale for continuous use of oral contraceptives', *Contraception*, vol. 74, no. 5, 2006, pp. 361–362. Archer, a clinical researcher at Eastern Virginia Medical School, points out that today pregnancy testing is readily available, accurate and inexpensive, thus removing the role of the visible withdrawal bleed.

35   Elsimar M. Coutinho with Sheldon J. Segal, *Is Menstruation Obsolete?* Oxford University Press, New York, 1999, pp. 5–8. See also Archer (2006), pp. 361–362.
36   Sarah L. Thomas, Charlotte Ellertson. 'Nuisance or natural and healthy: should monthly menstruation be optional for women?' *Lancet*, vol. 355, no. 9207, 11 March 2000, p. 923. The authors are researchers in women's reproductive health for the Population Council, Mexico.
37   Wyeth Pharmaceuticals funded a study on women's thoughts about menstrual suppression that involved surveying 1000 women in Brazil. See Emilia Sanabria, 'The politics of menstrual suppression in Brazil', *Anthropology News*, vol. 50, no. 2, 2009, p. 6.
38   Ingrid Johnston-Robledo, Jessica Barnack, Stephanie Wares, '"Kiss your period goodbye": menstrual suppression in the popular press', *Sex Roles*, vol. 54, nos. 5–6, 2006, p. 358.
39   Ingrid Johnston-Robledo, Melissa Ball, Kimberley Lauta and Ann Zekoll, 'To bleed or not to bleed: young women's attitudes toward menstrual suppression', *Women and Health*, vol. 38, no. 3, 2003, pp. 70–72. The authors are US psychologists. See also Linda C. Andrist, Alex Hoyt, Dawn Weinstein, Chris McGibbon, 'The need to bleed: women's attitudes and beliefs about menstrual suppression', *Journal of the American Academy of Nurse Practitioners*, vol. 16, no. 1, 2004, p. 35; and US psychologists Rose et al (2008), p. 698.

and the cleanser of toxic waste, contests the potential desirability of total menstrual suppression.[40]

One area in which menstrual suppression remains most controversial, both medically and socially, is that of the young non-sexually active girl, although there are indications that this is changing through second-generation familiarity with the Pill. Gynaecologist Andrew M. Kaunitz identifies two advantages to suppressing menstruation. The first is the benefit to bone health offered by reduction of blood loss, hence of iron-deficient anaemia, resulting in improved sporting activity levels and fewer musculoskeletal injuries. The second is that girls with earlier menarche will have less absenteeism from school due to painful periods, and be able to participate more in school activities. Kaunitz points out that many US doctors are now prescribing oral contraceptive pill regimes for young non-sexually active girls to regulate their menstrual cycles and reduce discomfort, and he recommends that doctors in general be confident about informing young girls and their mothers of the improved quality of life that menstrual suppression provides.[41] Furthermore, it is suggested by US paediatrician Ellen Rome that medical practitioners prescribe a monophasic monthly pack, with its equal quantities of oestrogen and progesterone, for young girls, instructing them to ignore the placebo pills and continue the active pills for up to 84 days. This particular regime reduces the incidence of spotting or bleeding, while allowing girls the convenience of choice in the timing of their pseudo-period during the last week or so.[42] However, menstrual manipulation in the young is not without certain risks. One being that social acceptance of it may lead to use by increasingly younger girls influenced by negative attitudes to the menstrual process or who simply do not want to have periods. The other concern is the effect on reproductive health, which menstrual cycle researcher, Christine Hitchcock, contends has

---

40   Simone Ferrero, Luiza Helena Abbamonte, Margherita Giordano, Franco Allessandri, Paola Anserini, Valentino Remorigida, Nicola Ragni, 'What is the desired menstrual frequency of women without menstrual-related symptoms?', *Contraception*, vol. 73, no. 5, 2006, pp. 537, 540. The authors are from the department of obstetrics and gynaecology, San Martino Hospital and the University of Genoa. See also Maria Clara Estanislau do Amaral, Ellen Hardy, Eliana Maria Hebling, Anibal Faúndes, 'Menstruation and amenorrhea: opinion of Brazilian women', *Contraception*, vol. 72, no. 2, 2005, pp. 158–159. Amenorrhea is the absence of menstruation. The authors are from the faculty of medical sciences, San Paulo. Do Amaral and Hardy are nurses and Hebling and Faúndes obstetricians and gynaecologists.

41   Andrew M. Kaunitz, 'Menstruation: choosing whether ... and when', *Contraception*, vol. 62, no. 6, 2000, pp. 280–281.

42   Caitlin W. Hicks and Ellen S, Rome, 'Menstrual manipulation: options for suppressing the cycle', *Cleveland Clinic Journal of Medicine*, vol. 77, no. 7, 2010, p. 447.

not yet been adequately assessed and is due to continuous oral contraceptive use having an increasingly suppressive effect on the hypothalamic-pituitary axis during the 12 or so years after menarche when the endocrine system is still developing.[43]

Nonetheless, oral contraceptives as menstrual suppressants are widely used with the introduction of the extended cycle oral contraception (ECOC), a 12-week cycle of 84 oral contraceptive pills and a seven-day placebo pill regime, providing four periods a year, and approved by the US Food and Drug Administration (FDA) in 2003.[44] Currently manufactured by different pharmaceutical companies and trade-named Seasonale and Seasonique, their difference is in the seven pills to cause withdrawal bleeding.[45] Seasonique contains minute quantities of synthesised oestrogen, ethinyl estradiol, to reduce second cycle spotting.[46] Prescribing information published by the manufacturer states that 12-month clinical trials indicated Seasonique is both safe and effective for use by women of reproductive age, but is only *expected* to be the same for post-pubescent girls under the age of 18 years, and not indicated for use in girls who have not reached menarche.[47] There is little doubt that the manufacturers believe their product is the way of the future for women because the first 365-day active pill regime with no placebo pills, trade-named Lybrel, was approved in the US by the FDA in May 2007, with applications made for the European Union market and for Australia and Canada with Lybrel trade-named Anya.[48] In the interim a study was made to evaluate the effect of current contraceptive practices on menstrual frequency among Australian university students, resulting in public health researchers calling

---

43   Christine L. Hitchcock, 'Elements of the menstrual suppression debate', *Health Care for Women International*, vol. 29, no. 7, 2008, pp. 710–711.

44   Jessica Shipman Gunson, '"More natural but less normal": reconsidering medicalisation and agency through women's accounts of menstrual suppression', *Social Science and Medicine*, vol. 71, no. 7, 2010, p. 1324. Gunson is a sociologist.

45   Anita L. Nelson and Lawrence S. Neinstein, 'Combination hormonal contraceptives', in Lawrence S. Neinstein, Catherine M. Gordon, Debra K. Katzman, David S. Rosen and Elizabeth R. Woods (eds), *Adolescent Health Care: a Practical Guide* (1984), fifth edition, Lippincott Williams and Wilkins, Philadelphia 2008, p. 597. Nelson is professor of obstetrics and gynaecology and Neinstein associate professor of paediatrics, both at UCLA.

46   Hicks and Rome (2010), p. 447. See also Nelson and Neinstein (2008), p. 597.

47   Prescribing information, *Seasonique*, http://www.seasonique.com/docs/prescribing-information.pdf, July 2010. Clinical studies were carried out with diverse groups of women including Caucasian 80%, African-American 11%, Hispanic 5%, Asian 2% and other 2%.

48   Nelson and Neinstein (2008), p. 597. See also Hitchcock (2008), p. 704.

for medical re-evaluation of extended-use oral contraception by young women.[49] Subsequently in 2012 an application for registration of the first ECOC, trade-name Yaz Flex, was approved by the Australian Therapeutic Goods Administration (TGA) and the drug became available by medical prescription. The active ingredients are ethinyloestradiol and a newer form of progesterone, drospirenone, which, according to some studies, is associated with an increased risk of venous thrombosis among women using ECOC. Nor is Yaz Flex to be used prior to menarche. The 120 pills come with a special dispenser allowing the user to read the status of intake, and consumer information advises a four-day break between extended cycles, reducing periods to three a year.[50]

Yet, as journalist Shelley Gare reports in an article titled 'Secret Women's Business', Family Planning Australia has been instructing women in menstrual suppression since the 1980s. Gare interviewed two women doctors, finding that young women are increasingly suppressing their periods. Dr Terri Foran, a sexual health physician and past director of Family Planning in NSW, estimates a quarter of young women attending her clinic use the pill to suppress bleeding. In Melbourne at the Jean Hailes Foundation for Women's Health, Dr Elizabeth Farrell observes an increase in menstrual suppression over the past decade, with more information about it being sought by teenagers and younger women. Farrell finds an association between menstrual suppression and the current social trends practised by teenagers and young women of total body epilation, and a demand for vaginal dryness, the latter regardless of explanation of purpose. She conjectures that having a period every month may become as gross as having hairy legs.[51]

We have seen the association between teenagers and menstrual suppression and the media and medical influences, both arguing social and educational benefits, and there are other groups also expressing the desirability of being free from menstrual bleeding. They include military service women deployed

---

49 Jessica Shipman Gunson (2010), p. 1327; Alecia J. Greig, Michelle A. Palmer, Lynne M. Chepulis, 'Hormonal contraceptive practices in young Australian women (<25 years) and their possible impact on menstrual frequency and iron requirements', *Sexual and Reproductive Healthcare*, vol. 1, no. 3, 2010, pp. 99–102. The participants were from Griffith University, Gold Coast campus.

50 Yaz Flex 'Public Summary' and 'Consumer Medicine Information', Therapeutic Goods Administration (Aust) www.tga.gov.au/file/6491/download; 'Product news', *Australian Pharmacist*, December 2012, pp. 990–91; Sue Dunlevy, 'New Pill adds comfort for women', Daily Telegraph, 25 September 2012; Deborah Bateson, 'What's new in contraception?' *O&G Magazine*, Vol. 14, no. 2, 2012, pp. 55–56.

51 Gare (2010), p. 51.

in a hostile environment.[52] Among currently deployed women in the US military there is support for menstrual suppression because of the benefits gained by freedom from stress-related menstrual irregularities and other related health problems and from menstrual hygiene difficulties. The ready availability of continuous use oral contraceptives from medical clinics during deployment, compared with variable supplies of menstrual hygiene products, indicates US military approval of the practice.[53] In civilian life women engaging in athletics who wish to eliminate bleeding and preserve bone health are using ECOC[54] and an Italian study shows women's preferences for varying durations of menstrual suppression as a means of improving their lives in the workplace, in clothing choice, in sporting activities and in sexual activity.[55] Similar evidence gathered internationally indicates that women in industrialised countries prefer less bleeding for reasons of convenience.[56]

Convenience plays a part in women's lives but long or extended-cycle oral contraception require women to remember to take a daily pill. An alternative is the injectable synthesised progesterone derivative, depot medroxyproges-terone acetate (DMPA), given the trade name Depo Provera. The drug, initially intended to prevent late-term miscarriage and premature labour in women, failed its trials in Brazil under the supervision of Dr Elsimar Coutinho, but unexpectedly produced evidence of ovulatory suppression with accompanying menstrual suppression, lasting up to six months follow-ing treatment. Cessation of Depo Provera allowed ovulation to resume, and pregnancy to occur, and during the time of menstrual suppression Coutinho found evidence of improved health in women with pre-existing anaemia, associated with higher resistance to disease and greater stamina due to increased levels of iron, hence haemoglobin or red blood cells. Moreover, women recognised the benefits of not menstruating.[57]

---

52 Diane Wind Wardell and Barbara Czerwinski, 'A military challenge to managing feminine and personal hygiene', *Journal of the American Academy of Nurse Practitioners*, vol. 13, no. 4, 2001, pp. 187–188. Wardell is professor of nursing at the University of Texas and Czerwinski is director of emergency room nursing at Ben Taub Hospital, Texas.

53 Lori L. Trego and Patricia J. Jordan, 'Military women's attitudes toward menstruation and menstrual suppression in relation to the deployed environment', *Women's Health Issues*, vol. 20, no. 4, 2010, pp. 291–292. Trego is a US army nurse and Jordan is a US research methodologist.

54 David F. Archer, 'Menstrual-cycle related symptoms: a review of the rationale for continuous use of oral contraceptives', *Contraception*, vol. 74, no. 5, 2006, p. 364.

55 Ferrero et al (2006), p. 539.

56 I. Wiegratz, H.H. Hommel, T. Zimmermann, H. Kuhl, 'Attitude of German women and gynaecologists towards long-cycle treatment with oral contraceptives', *Contraception*, vol. 69, no. 1, 2004, p. 41. The authors are gynaecologists.

57 Coutinho (1999), pp. 8–11, 117–118.

Having refuted the belief that menstrual suppression contravenes a law of nature, Coutinho insists that beliefs in the benefits of menstruation to women have no grounding in scientific evidence, but that menstruation exists only as a consequence of the process of reproduction.[58] He argues the benefit of menstrual suppression in countries where early menarche is followed by pregnancy, drawing attention to the situation in the US where young girls of 10–14 years contribute some 12,000 babies to the statistics of babies born annually to children, and that in 1995 about 30,000 girls in Brazil, aged 10–11 years-old, became pregnant, many to family members. Thus, by impeding early menarche by delaying the hormonal activation of ovulation and slowing down sexual development, girls are given several additional menstruation-free years while reducing the risk of assault to the prematurely maturing body.[59]

Depo Provera, approved for contraceptive use in 1992 and available worldwide, is administered by four injections annually, allowing women the choice of remaining both pregnancy and menstruation-free.[60] An information sheet about the drug, provided by the Royal Women's Hospital, Melbourne, points out that women need to remember the injections must be repeated on 12-weekly basis for Depo Provera to remain effective. Women are also cautioned to think about the non-reversibility of the drug once the injection has been administered.[61] The negative effects of any drug on bone health is a matter for concern, and in 2006 WHO issued a statement on depot medroxyprogesterone acetate (DMPA), Depo Provera, showing evidence of some effect on bone mineral density (BMD) in certain women and in adolescents who have not reached optimal bone mass. Results are variable and indicate that in girls from menarche to 18 years there is a loss of about 5–7 per cent after two years' continual use of the drug, equating to that in lactating women, however the rate of loss appears to decrease over time and bone mineral density increases when the drug is ceased. WHO recommends that no restriction be imposed on the use of DPMA for adolescents from menarche to 18 years of age because the advantages of the drug outweigh the

---

58   Coutinho (1999), p. 163.
59   Coutinho (1999), pp. 114, 162–163. The Australian figures for girls 15–19 years, which include girls less than 15 years, were 12,120 births in 2009. The pre Depo Provera figure for 1989 was 14,259 and this reduced to 12,853 in 1994 according to the Australian Bureau of Statistics: 301.0: Births, Australia, 2009. Summary tables: 2.20 Births, Australia – selected years at http://www.abs.gov.au/ausstats/abs@nsf/Products/5ECFEOF9C48
60   Coutinho (1999), pp. 10, 117–118. He draws attention to the availability of several other oral or vaginal progestins that can produce the same effect as Depo Provera.
61   'Depo Provera: a contraceptive injection', http://www.thewomens.org.au/DepoProveraAContraceptiveInjection

risks of bone fracture, however, lack of data with long-term users indicates reconsideration of use with individuals over time.[62]

Both the long or extended cycle oral contraceptive and the injectable depot medroxyprogesterone acetate have provided women in developed countries with choices and mechanisms of control over their fertility and their menstrual cycles. The negative aspects of side effects and remaining concerns felt by some women about issues of safety have not reduced the continuing interest in, and use of, these drugs, which are expected to be increasingly available in developing countries and promoted through the media.[63]

The extent to which menstrual suppression will be a choice for young women in developing countries is unclear due to several reasons. Women, particularly those in remote areas, are not accustomed to regular regimes of pill-taking or injections and their lack of education prevents them fully understanding information given about hormone-altering drugs and their side effects. Nor is it clear whether health workers will be adequately knowledgeable to instruct in these matters. The relationship between pharmaceutical companies and governments regarding distribution of menstrual suppressant drugs may also be based on state population control programs with few checks and balances protecting young women users.[64] Nevertheless young women of the future will re-think menstrual practice in the knowledge of their world. There are strong indications that menstrual suppression will be part of the choices they make, although the historian Sharra Vostral argues that long-term menstrual suppression causes women to become estranged from their bodies and lose the cultural meanings attributed to menstruation.[65] Thus, women in developed countries are no longer defined by their reproductive potential but by the skills and abilities that enable them to carry out multiple aspects of social life.

Conclusion

The future of menarche appears dependent on two issues: women's education and the value society places on women as reproductive bodies. The historic influence of religious belief systems on control of the menstruating body,

---

62   Catherine d'Arcangues, 'WHO statement on hormonal contraception and bone health', *Contraception*, vol. 73, no. 5, 2006, pp. 443–444. D'Arcangues is a researcher in reproductive health for WHO.

63   Rose et al (2008), pp. 698–699.

64   Farida Akhter, 'The state of contraceptive technology in Bangladesh', *Reproductive and Genetic Engineering*, vol. 1, no. 2, 1988, pp. 159–161.

65   Sharra L. Vostral, *Under Wraps: a History of Menstrual Hygiene Technology*, Lexingham Books, Lanham, Maryland 2008, p. 171.

hence the sexuality of women, has been weakened in developed countries as a result of change in social values paralleling scientific and technological advancement which has advanced medical thought and practice. One result is that girls now reach menarche with the expectation of a future career, geographic mobility, continuous electronic communication and some knowledge of the existence of control over their fertility. Advancements in knowledge of women's hormone function has enabled women to control menstruation and there is increased interest by post-menarcheal girls in menstrual suppression, a practice with positive and negative benefits under medical debate, as we have seen.

In developing countries the future of menarche is less clear. Change in cultural traditions and practices are slow and uneven, and many girls are still struggling to receive an education in societies where women are valued primarily for their reproductive body. Although interview data with Indian women indicates a diminishing cultural tradition of menstrual seclusion within urban, educated, families, several interviewees referred to its continuation among the poor and uneducated who also maintain the dowry tradition. However, it is significant that a number of the information sources used for reference in this chapter reflect educated Indian and African women's association with NGOs, and their involvement with menstrual hygiene education and practice at village level. The formation of women's cooperatives, including participation in local or regional manufacture and distribution of inexpensive disposable menstrual absorbents, has improved women's menstrual health, but at an environmental cost caused by menstrual waste, a concern absent from my interview data, but one with increasing significance for the future. The acceptance of menstrual suppression by women in developing countries, while potentially beneficial physically and environmentally, contests the value associated with the menstrual evidence of their reproductive body.

Nonetheless, scientific and technological developments will continue to define the future of menarche as the starting point of a range of practices relating to menstrual life, extending from hygienic management to its complete avoidance.

CONCLUSION

This book has been a journey of exploration built around the key argument that although menarche is a shared physiological experience in the lives of pubescent girls, the meanings associated with it have been constructed from antiquity through the continuing influences of medicine and religion. These influences, generated in patriarchal societies, have dominated and reinforced cultural ideas of control of women's bodies, symbolised through the control of menstruation beginning at the signal moment of menarche. Further investigation indicates how traditional thought and practice relating to menarche and menstruation are being displaced by a widening science-based knowledge resulting in different perceptions of what cyclical bleeding means in women's lives today.

Initially I had expected that interview data would indicate considerable cultural variation in meanings associated with menarche, and that there would be a diversity of women who had begun menstrual life with ceremony, further emphasising cultural variation. Neither expectation was fully met. My interview data confirmed that for the majority of interviewees the cultural meanings associated with menarche came from medicine, shaping certain cultural similarities, and giving evidence of the endurance of ancient medical thought in both Eastern and Western traditions about young women's bodies. Endurance of ancient thought was revealed also through reference to ideas and comments from the writing of Pliny the Elder, the Classical Roman naturalist and philosopher, which were heard in beliefs about women's blood spoken of by a number of my interviewees.

In a similar way, the historical influence of religious belief systems on matters of women's bodies and blood follows the written tenets of the major world religions. One example commonly heard among interviewees was that of 'becoming unclean', an ancient explanation of the anomaly of a girl's body bleeding unexpectedly, then cyclically, in the absence of disease or injury. The concept was explored further through a closer examination of the menstrual practices prescribed by religious law, including menstrual taboo and seclusion from the time of menarche, and through identifying changes in religious thought toward menstruation.

Before culturally conventional meanings are transmitted to the young girl at menarche, there is usually a lone moment of discovery. This was remembered by interviewees in two ways: acceptance and terror. Some spoke of being alienated from a body that had suddenly become unreliable, resulting in menarche being the site of a struggle for control. Others related how menarche forced upon them a decision to become independent and to keep the knowledge of bleeding to themselves. Emotional maturity was shown to be a significant factor in whether the menarcheal experience was positive or negative, and the adolescent concept of the social clock, registering personal progress within the peer group, was seen to work positively when menarche was on time, but have a negative effect where deviance caused by prematurity had occurred.

Underlying the influence of the formal medical and religious teachings about menarche and menstruation is a parallel body of informal knowledge, women's lore, often referred to as 'old wives' tales'. This is an oral repository maintained by older women and transmitted at times of life events such as menarche. Several interviewees remembered receiving instructions that took three definable forms involving bodily power, vulnerability, and methods of controlling the menstrual body. Women's lore has a mythical quality resonating with some past event and remains of interest to folklore exponents, although its disappearance reflects wider educational opportunities for women at a time when scientific research has indicated the presence of some validity among the tales.

Another disappearing experience associated with menarche is the ceremony, which remains of considerable importance in many cultures – in the introduction to the thesis I described my impressions of the Apache puberty ceremony. I had hoped this would be a prelude to learning more about this aspect of cultural diversity, but unfortunately very few interviewees had gone through a menarche ceremony. Three Sri Lankan women recalled their experiences, one explaining the importance of giving her Australian-born daughter a menarche ceremony as a cultural link with the girl's Sri Lankan heritage. None of the Indian interviewees had experienced the transitional formality, although there was a general awareness of the custom. A Fijian woman had witnessed her older sister's menarche ceremony and described her childhood memory of it; and a Javanese woman reminisced about a flower-adorned ritual bath. The events recalled by interviewees were placed in a framework suggested by Arnold van Gennep's theory on rites of passage through the major transitions of life. This enabled me to argue the way in which menarche ceremonies evolved to other forms in modern societies.

The evolution of medical research and technology and increased financial enterprise played a role in constructing meaning in the unique biological process we know as menarche. Thus 20th-century economics may be argued to be the third and possibly most powerful influence on the way we now think of women's bodies and blood. The seemingly universal need for freedom from the stigma of revealed menstrual blood, and the ways in which young women achieved it, were frequently spoken of throughout the interviews, confirming the link between women's freedom, physically and socially, and effective menstrual absorbents. There was little doubt that the availability of modern disposable pads and tampons came to determine the meanings that women constructed about their periods from the time of menarche. Women and girls became willing consumers, with certain medical and social consequences.

In the US, women's acceptance of disposable menstrual absorbents led to the manufacturing companies developing menstrual education programs for girls, under the direction of medical practitioners, which expanded into other countries including Australia. Thus commercial interests appropriated the traditionally maternal role which had frequently resulted in more ignorance rather than enlightenment. Distribution of this knowledge was made privately through booklets and publicly through selected schools by talks, films and product information and hand-outs in an ongoing promotion intended to create loyal consumerism throughout menstrual life. This was remembered by interviewees in Singapore and the Philippines.

Today, menarche is shadowed by complex technologies. Soon after the event many young women in the West are increasingly considering available methods to suppress menstruation, a pattern that may be adopted by young women in developing countries. In the West there is familiarity with the concept of oral contraception, the perception of availability, safety and reversibility of effects, with the principal sources of information being friends, the media and medical practitioners. However, an overall knowledge of the menstrual cycle remains somewhat limited. In developing countries, women's choice in the use of continuous oral or injectable contraception and menstrual suppression may be dictated by wealth, or poverty, and will depend on how their nation's government and non-government org-anisations perceive national advantages and disadvantages in the context of reproductive health, environmental concerns and workplace labour.

The influences bringing about change in cultural meanings associated with menarche had traditionally been associated with men until women gained access to educational opportunities. Since the advent of modern dis-posable sanitary absorbents, women have taken an increasingly influential role in issues relating to menarche and menstruation, initially as advisers, product promoters and educators on behalf of the manufacturing companies.

Women drove the search for oral contraception. Women have conducted later evaluative studies into continuous oral contraception; women medical practitioners are consultants on menstrual and reproductive health; women publish articles on menstrual options in popular journals. In developing countries the older women, who uphold traditional beliefs on menstrual seclusion, are being educated with their daughters in matters of menstrual hygiene and health. Their teachers demonstrate a working relationship with men, breaking cultural silence on the subject at both government and village levels. In other words, women are changing the ways in which meanings about menarche and menstruation, constructed by men, have traditionally been maintained, but it is women, too, who manipulated them for their own purposes, and so it is today in the West with technology such as the Pill. In remote areas of developing nations, where women's physical labour is hard, the rest afforded them by menstrual seclusion may be beneficial, but it is a situation requiring compliance until cultural change renders it obsolete. Meanwhile women are involved in changing how we think about menarche and menstruation. That is, they are changing cultural constructs. They are reclaiming their bodies and they are appropriating scientific knowledge to help them determine how and when they menstruate.

BIBLIOGRAPHY

Books

Antonelli, Judith S., *In the Image of God: a Feminist Commentary on the Torah*, Jason Aronson Inc., New Jersey, 1995

Aristotle, *Generation of Animals, XIII*, trans. A. L. Peck (1942), Loeb Classical Library, William Heinemann Limited, London, 1963

Attwood, Bain, *Possession: Batman's Treaty and the Matter of History*, Miegunyah Press, Carlton, 2009

Bede, *A History of the English Church and People*, trans. Leo Shirley-Price, Penguin, Middlesex, 1956

Bell, Catherine M., *Ritual: Perspectives and Dimensions*, Oxford University Press, New York, 1997

Beyene, Yewoubdar, *From Menarche to Menopause: Reproductive Lives of Peasant Women in Two Cultures*, State University of New York Press, Albany, 1989

Bloch, Abraham P., *The Biblical and Historical Background of Jewish Customs and Ceremonies*, Ktav Publishing House Inc., New York, 1980

The Book of Common Prayer (1662), Oxford University Press, London n.d., c. 1950

Chamberlain, Mary, *Old Wives' Tales: Their History, Remedies and Spells*, Virago Press Limited, London, 1981

Cohen, Paul A., *History in Three Keys: the Boxers as Event, Experience, and Myth*, Columbia University Press, New York, 1997

Coutinho, Elsimar M., with Segal, Sheldon J., *Is Menstruation Obsolete?* Oxford University Press, New York, 1999

Dean-Jones, Lesley, *Women's Bodies in Classical Greek Science*, (1994) Oxford University Press, Oxford, 2001

Delaney, Janice, Lupton, Mary Jane, Toth, Emily, *The Curse: a Cultural History of Menstruation* (1976), revised edition, University of Illinois Press, Urbana, 1988

Demand, Nancy H., *Birth, Death and Motherhood in Classical Greece*, The Johns Hopkins University Press, Baltimore, 1994

Douglas, Mary, *Purity and Danger: an Analysis of Concept of Pollution and Taboo* (1966), Routledge Classics, London, 2008

Dundes, Alan, *Folklore matters*, The University of Tennessee Press, Knoxville, 1989

Farrer, Claire R., *Living Life's Circle: Mescalero Apache Cosmovision*, University of New Mexico Press, Albuquerque, 1991

Faure, Bernard, *The Power of Denial: Buddhism, Purity, and Gender*, Princeton University Press, New Jersey, 2003

Fonrobert, Charlotte Elisheva, *Menstrual Purity: Rabbinic and Christian Reconstructions of Biblical Gender*, Stanford, California, 2000

Fothergill, W. E., *Manual of Midwifery for the use of Students and Practitioners*, William F. Clay, Edinburgh, 1903

Foucault, Michel, *The Birth of the Clinic: an Archaeology of Medical Perception*, trans. M. Sheridan Smith, Vintage Books, New York, 1994

Frazer, James George, *The Golden Bough: a Study in Magic and Religion*, (1890), abridged edition, vol. II (1922), Macmillan and Company Limited, London, 1957

Furth, Charlotte, *A Flourishing Yin: Gender in China's Medical History, 960–1665*, University of California Press, Berkeley and Los Angeles, 1999

Geertz, Clifford, *The Interpretation of Cultures*, Basic Books, New York, 1973

Hewitt, Graily, *The Pathology, Diagnosis, and Treatment of the Diseases of Women*, fourth edition, Longmans, Green, and Company, London, 1882

Kapadia, Karin, *Siva and her Sisters: Gender, Caste, and Class in Rural South India*, Westview Press, Boulder, 1995

Kaptchuk, Ted J. *Chinese Medicine: the Web that has no Weaver* (1983), Rider and Company, Essex, 1987

King, Helen, *Hippocrates' Woman: Reading the Female Body in Ancient Greece*, Routledge, London, 1998

Lee, Janet, and Sasser-Coen, Jennifer, *Blood Stories: Menarche and the Politics of the Female Body in Contemporary U.S. Society*, Routledge, New York, 1996

Levy, Robert I., *Tahitians: Mind and Experience in the Society Islands*, University of Chicago Press, Chicago, 1973

Marcus, Ivan G., *The Jewish Life Cycle: Rites of Passage from Biblical to Modern Times*, University of Washington Press, Seattle, 2004

McCalman, Janet, *Journeyings: The Biography of a Middle-Class Generation 1920–1990* (1993), Melbourne University Press, Carlton, 1995

McCalman, Janet, *Sex and Suffering: Women's Health and a Women's Hospital*, Melbourne University Press, Melbourne, 1998

McQuarrie, John, *A Guide to the Sacraments*, Continuum, New York, 1999

Melendy, Mary R., *Perfect Womanhood for Maidens – Wives – Mothers*, World Publishing Company, Guelph, Ontario, 1901

Mernissi, Fatima, *Women and Islam: an Historical and Theological Enquiry*, trans. Mary Jo Lakeland, Women Unlimited Press, New Delhi, 2004

Morton, Helen, *Becoming Tongan: an Ethnography of Childhood*, University of Hawai'I Press, Honolulu, 1996

Myles, Margaret F., *Textbook for Midwives*, Churchill Livingstone, Edinburgh, 1975

Opler, Morris E., *An Apache Life-Way: the Economic, Social, and Religious Institutions of the Chiricahua Indians* (1941), Cooper Square Publishers Inc., New York, 1965

Paige, Karen Ericksen, and Paige, Jeffrey M., *The Politics of Reproductive Ritual*, University of California Press, Berkeley, 1981

Pliny, *Natural History with an English Translation in Ten Volumes, Vol. VIII*, trans. W.H.S. Jones, William Heinemann Limited, London, 1963

Radaza, Francisco Demetrio y, S. J. (comp. and ed.), *Dictionary of Philippine Folk Beliefs and Customs, Book II and Book III*, Xavier University, Cagayan de Oro City, 1970

Rasing, Thera, *Passing on the Rites of Passage: Girls' Initiation Rites in the Context of an Urban Roman Catholic Community on the Zambian Copperbelt*, African Studies Centre, Leiden University Research Series 6, Amsterdam, 1995

Ross, Mandy, *Coming of Age*, Heinemann Library, Oxford, 2003

Sarkar, Tanika, *Hindu Wife, Hindu Nation: Community, Religion, and Cultural Nationalism*, Indiana University Press, Bloomington, Indiana, 2001

Seymour-Smith, Charlotte, *Macmillan Dictionary of Anthropology* (1986), The Macmillan Press, London, 1993

The Shorter Oxford English Dictionary, third edition, 1944, C. T. Onions (ed.), Oxford, 1959

Showalter, Elaine, *The Female Malady: Women, Madness, and English Culture, 1830–1980*, Penguin Books, New York, 1987

Singer, Charles, *From Magic to Science*, Dover Publications, New York, 1958

Smith, David, *Hinduism and Modernity*, Blackwell Publishing, Oxford, 2003

Soranus, *Gynaecology*, trans. Owsei Temkin (1956), Johns Hopkins University Press, Baltimore, 1991

Stockel, H. Henrietta, *Chiricahua Apache Women and Children: Safekeepers of the Heritage*, Texas A&M University Press, College Station, 2000

Summers, Anne, *Damned Whores and God's Police*, second revised edition, Penguin Books, Camberwell, 2002

Trotula, *The Trotula: a Medieval Compendium of Women's Medicine*, trans. Monica H. Green (ed.), University of Pennsylvania Press, Philadelphia, 2001

Unschuld, Paul U., *Huang Di nei jing su wen: Nature, Knowledge, Imagery in an Ancient Chinese Medical Text*, University of California Press, Berkeley and Los Angeles, 2003

Vansina, Jan, *Oral Tradition: a Study in Historical Methodology*, trans. H.M. Wright, Routledge and Keegan Paul, London, 1969

Van Gennep, Arnold, *The Rites of Passage* (1908), trans. Monika B. Vizedom and Gabrielle L. Caffee, University of Chicago Press, Chicago, 1960

Vostral, Sharra L., *Under Wraps: a History of Menstrual Hygiene Technology*, Lexington Books, Lanham, Maryland, 2008

Walker, Benjamin, *Hindu World: an Encyclopaedic Survey of Hinduism*, Indus Press, New Delhi, 1995

Watson, J. K., *A Complete Handbook of Midwifery for Midwives and Nurses*, The Scientific Press Limited, London, 1904

Whittaker, Andrea, *Intimate Knowledge: Women and their Health in North-East Thailand*, Allen and Unwin, St Leonards, NSW, 2000

Wickremeratne, Swarna, *Buddhism in Sri Lanka: Remembered Yesterdays*, State University of New York Press, Albany, 2006

Wujastyk, Dominik, *The Roots of Ayurveda* (1998), including the author's translations of Suśruta's *Compendium* and Kaśyapa's *Compendium*, Penguin Books Limited, London, 2003

Chapters in Books

Andresen, Rhonda, 'Hawai'i', in *Narratives and Images of Pacific Island Women*, Debbie Hippolite Wright, Rosalind Meno Ram, and Kathleen Fromm Ward (eds), Women's Studies, Volume 44, The Edwin Mellen Press, Lewiston, New York, 2005

Arata, Luigi, 'Menses in the corpus Hippocraticum', in *Menstruation: a Cultural History*, Andrew Shail and Gillian Howie (eds), Palgrove Macmillan, Basingstoke, 2005

Bechert, Heinz, 'Remarks on astrological sanskrit literature from Sri Lanka', in *Senarat Paranavitana Commemoration Volume, vol. 7*, Leelananda Prematilleke, Karthigesu Indrapala and J. E. van Lohizen-de Leeuw (eds), composed by Sri Lanka Press, Leiden, The Netherlands, 1978

Blackman, Helen, 'Embryological and agricultural constructions of the menstrual cycle, 1890–1910, in *Menstruation: a Cultural History*, Andrew Shail and Gillian Howie (eds), Palgrave Macmillan, Basingstoke, 2005

Buckley, Thomas, Gottlieb, Alma, 'A critical appraisal of the theories of menstrual symbolism', in *Blood Magic: the Anthropology of Menstruation*, Thomas Buckley and Alma Gottlieb (eds), University of California Press, Berkeley, 1988

Edmonds, D. Keith, 'Gynaecological disorders of childhood and adolescence', in *Dewhursts's Textbook of Obstetrics and Gynaecology*, D. Keith Edmonds and John Dewhurst (eds), seventh edition, Wiley-Blackwell Publishing, Oxford, 2007

'Genesis', in *The Holy Bible*, King James' version, Cambridge University Press, Cambridge n.d.

Gottlieb, Alma, 'Menstrual cosmology among the Beng of Ivory Coast', in *Blood Magic: the Anthropology of Menstruation*, Thomas Buckley and Alma Gottlieb (eds), University of California Press, Berkeley, 1988

Green, Monica H., 'Flowers, poisons and men: menstruation in medieval Western Europe', in *Menstruation: a Cultural History*, Andrew Shail, Gillian Howie (eds), Palgrove Macmillan, Basingstoke, 2005

Gross, Rita, 'Buddhism', in *Her Voice, Her Faith: Women Speak Out on World Religions*, Arvind Sharma, Katherine K. Young (eds), Westview Press, Cambridge, Maryland, 2002

Hippocrates, 'Girls', in *Hippocrates Vol. IX*, trans. Paul Potter (ed.), Loeb Classical Library, Harvard University Press, Cambridge (US), 2010

Hull, Terence H., and Hull, Valerie J., 'Means, motives and menses: use of herbal emmenagogues in Indonesia', in *Regulating Menstruation: Beliefs, Practices, Interpretations*, Etienne Van de Walle, and Elisha P. Renne (eds), University of Chicago Press, Chicago, 2001

'Isaiah', in *The Holy Bible*, King James' version, Cambridge University Press, Cambridge, n.d.

Kimball, Solon T., 'Introduction' to Arnold Van Gennep, *Rites of Passage*, trans. Monika B. Vizedom and Gabrielle L. Caffee, University of Chicago Press, Chicago, 1960

Lainer, Ilene, 'The Slap, 1972', in *My Little Red Book*, Rachel Kauder Nalebuff (ed.), Twelve, New York, 2009

Lake, Marilyn, 'Freedom, fear and the family', in Patricia Grimshaw, Marilyn Lake, Ann McGrath, Marian Quartly, *Creating a Nation*, McPhee Gribble Publishers, Penguin Books, Ringwood, 1994

Lawrence, Denise L., 'Menstrual politics: women and pigs in rural Portugal', in *Blood Magic: the Anthropology of Menstruation*, Thomas Buckley and Alma Gottlieb (eds), University of California Press, Berkeley, 1988

Ledger, William L., 'The Menstrual Cycle', in *Dewhurst's Textbook of Obstetrics and Gynaecology*, D. Keith Edmonds and John Dewhurst (eds), seventh edition, Wiley-Blackwell Publishing, 2007

Leslie, Julia, 'Some traditional Indian views on menstruation and female sexuality', in *Sexual Knowledge, Sexual Science: the History of Attitudes to Sexuality*, Roy Porter and Mikuláš Teich (eds), Cambridge University Press, Cambridge, 1994

'Leviticus', in *The Holy Bible*, King James' version, Cambridge University Press, Cambridge n.d.

Loudon, Irving S. L., 'Childbirth', in *Companion Encyclopedia of the History of Medicine, Vol. 2*, W. F. Bynum and Roy Porter (eds) (1993), Routledge, London, 1997

Lutkehaus, Nancy C., 'Feminist anthropology and female initiation in Melanesia', in *Gender Rituals: Female Initiation in Melanesia*, Nancy Lutkehaus and Paul B. Roscoe (eds), Routledge, New York, 1995

Manaf, Nor Faridah Abdul, 'Other coming of age rituals among Malay Muslim girls in Malaysia', in *The Encyclopedia of Women and Islamic Cultures: Family, Body, Sexuality and Health, Vol. 3*, Suad Joseph and Afsaneh Najmabadi (eds), Koninklijke Brill NV, Leiden, The Netherlands, 2006

Maschio, Thomas, 'Mythic images and objects of myth in Rauto female puberty ritual' in *Gender Rituals: Female Initiation in Melanesia*, Nancy Lutkehaus and Paul B. Roscoe (eds), Routledge, New York, 1995

McClive, Cathy, 'Menstrual knowledge and medical practice in early modern France c. 1555–1761, in *Menstruation: a Cultural History*, Andrew Shail and Gillian Howie (eds), Palgrave Macmillan, Basingstoke, 2005

Milow, Vera J., 'Menstrual education: past, present and future', in *Menarche: the Transition from Girl to Woman*, Sharon Golub (ed.), Lexington Books, Lexington, 1983

Myerhoff, Barbara, 'Rites of passage: process and paradox', in *Celebration: Studies in Festivity and Ritual*, Victor Turner (ed.), Smithsonian Institution Press, Washington DC, 1982

Narayanan, Vasudha, 'Hinduism', in *Her Voice, Her Faith: Women Speak on World Religions*, Arvind Sharma and Katherine K. Young (eds), Westview Press, Cambridge, Maryland, 2002

Nelson, Anita L., and Neinstein,,Lawrence S., 'Combination hormonal contraceptives', in Lawrence S. Neinstein, Catherine M. Gordon, Debra K. Katzman, David S. Rosen and Elizabeth R. Woods (eds), *Adolescent Health Care: a Practical Guide* (1984), fifth edition, Lippincott Williams and Wilkins, Philadelphia, 2008

Ner-David, Haviva, 'Medieval *responsa* literature on Niddah: perpetuations of notions of *tumah*' in *Menstruation: a Cultural History*, Andrew Shail and Gillian Howie (eds), Palgrove Macmillan, Basingstoke, 2005

Niehof, Anke, 'Traditional medicine at pregnancy and childbirth in Madura, Indonesia' in *The Context of Medicines in Developing Countries: Studies in Pharmaceutical Anthropology*, Sjaak van der Geest and Susan Reynolds Whyte (eds), Kluwer Academic Publishers, Dordrecht, The Netherlands, 1988

Paige, Karen Ericksen, 'Social Aspects of Menstruation' in *Cultural Perspectives on Biological Knowledge*, Troy Duster and Karen Garrett (eds), Ablex Publishing Co., New Jersey, 1984

Parkin, David, 'Ritual as spatial direction and bodily division', in *Understanding Rituals*, Daniel de Coppet (ed.), Routledge, London, 1992

Phillips, Kim, 'Maidenhood as the perfect age of woman's life' in *Young Medieval Women*, Katherine J. Lewis, Noël James Menuge and Kim M. Phillips (eds), Sutton Publishing, Gloucestershire, 1999

Rackham, H., 'Introduction' in *Pliny: Natural History with an English Translation in Ten Volumes, Vol. I*, trans. H. Rackham, William Heinemann Limited, London, 1967

Reed, Barbara E., 'The gender symbolism of Kuan-yin bodhisattva', in *Buddhism, Sexuality, and Gender*, José Ignacio Cabezón (ed.), State University of New York Press, Albany, 1992

Sewell, William Jr., 'The concept(s) of culture' in *Beyond the Cultural Turn: New Directions on the Study of Society and Culture*, Victoria E. Bonnell and Lynn Hunt (eds), University of California Press, Berkeley, 1999

Showalter, Elaine, Showalter, English, 'Victorian women and menstruation' in *Suffer and be Still: Women in the Victorian Age*, Martha Vicinus (ed.), first published Indiana University Press, Bloomington, 1972. Second printing 1973

Sponberg, Alan, 'Attitudes toward women and the feminine in early Buddhism', in *Buddhism, Sexuality and Gender*, José Ignacio Cabezón (ed.), State University of New York Press, Albany, 1992

Suan, Mary, 'More islands' in *Narratives and Images of Pacific Island Women*, Debbie Hippolite Wright, Rosalind Meno Ram, Kathleen Fromm Ward (eds), Women's Studies, Volume 44, The Edwin Mellen Press, Lewiston, New York, 2005

Temkin, Owsei, 'Introduction', in *Soranus Gynaecology* (1965), trans. Owsei Temkin, The Johns Hopkins University Press, Baltimore, 1991

Wear, Andrew, 'The story of personal hygiene', in *Companion Encyclopedia of the History of Medicine*, vol. 2, W. F. Bynum and Roy Porter (eds), Routledge, London, 1997

Wilms, Sabine, 'The art and science of menstrual balancing in early medieval China', in *Menstruation: a Cultural History*, Andrew Shail and Gillian Howie (eds), Palgrove Macmillan, Basingstoke, 2005

Journal Articles

Akhter, Farida 'The state of contraceptive technology in Bangladesh', *Reproductive and Genetic Engineering*, vol. 1, no. 2, 1988

Al-Khalidi, Alia, 'Emergent technologies in menstrual paraphernalia in mid-nineteenth-century Britain', *Journal of Design History*, vol. 14, no. 4, 2001

Anderson, Elizabeth Garrett, 'Sex in mind and education: a reply', *Fortnightly Review*, vol. 15, no. 89, 1 May 1874

Andrist, Linda C., Hoyt, Alex, Weinstein, Dawn, McGibbon, Chris, 'The need to bleed: women's attitudes and beliefs about menstrual suppression', *Journal of the American Academy of Nurse Practitioners*, vol. 16, no. 1, 2004

Archer, David F., 'Menstrual-cycle-related symptoms: a review of the rationale for continuous use of oral contraceptives', *Contraception*, vol. 74, no. 5, 2006

Arnold, Lloyd, and Hagele, Marie, 'Vaginal tamponage for catamenial sanitary protection', *Journal of the American Medical Association*, vol. 110, no. 11, 1938

Ashley-Montagu, M. F., 'Physiology and the origin of the menstrual prohibitions', *The Quarterly Review of Biology*, vol. 15, no. 2, 1940

Author undisclosed, 'Reviews and notices of books', *Lancet*, vol. 103, no. 2645, 9 May 1874

Author undisclosed, 'The folklore of menstruation', *Lancet*, vol. 175, no. 4507, 15 January 1910

Barton, Mary, 'Review of the sanitary appliance with a discussion in intravaginal packs', *British Medical Journal*, vol. 1, no. 4243, 1942

Bateson, Deborah, 'What's new in contraception?' *O&G Magazine*, vol. 14, no. 2, 2012

Ben-Noun, Liubov (Louba), 'What is the biblical attitude towards personal hygiene during vaginal bleeding?' *European Journal of Obstetrics and Gynaecology and Reproductive Biology*, vol. 106, no. 1, 2003

Bradra, M., 'Changing age of marriage of girls in India', *International Journal of Anthropology*, vol. 15, nos 1-2, 2000

Brander, M. S., 'Tampons in menstruation' *British Medical Journal*, vol. 1, no. 4239, 1942

Britton, Cathryn J., 'Learning about "The Curse": an anthropological perspective on experiences of menstruation', *Women's Studies International Forum*, vol. 19, no. 6, 1996

Brookes, Barbara and Tennant, Margaret, 'Making girls modern: Pakeha women and menstruation in New Zealand 1930–70', *Women's History Review*, vol. 7, no. 4, 1998

Brown, Judith, 'A cross-cultural study of female initiation rites', *American Anthropologist*, vol. 65, no. 4, 1963

Brumberg, Joan Jacobs, '"Something happens to girls": menarche and the emergence of the modern American hygienic imperative', *Journal of the History of Sexuality*, vol. 4, no. 1, 1993

Bryant, J. A., Heathcote, D.G., Pickles, V. R., 'The search for "menotoxin"', *The Lancet*, vol. 309, issue 18014, 2 April 1977

Bullough, Vern L., 'Technology and female sexuality: some implications', *The Journal of Sex Research*, vol. 16, no. 1, 1980

Bullough, Vern L., 'Age at menarche: a misunderstanding', *Science*, New Series, vol. 213, no. 4505, 1981

Bullough, Vern L., 'Merchandising the sanitary napkin: Lilian Gilbreth's 1927 survey', *Signs*, vol. 10, no. 3, 1985

Cardwell, Mary G., 'Tampons in menstruation', *British Medical Journal*, vol.1, no. 4242, 1942

Chisholm, James S., Quinlivan, Julie A., Petersen, Rodney W., Coall, David A., 'Early stress predicts age at menarche and first birth, adult attachment, and expected lifespan', *Human Nature*, vol. 16, no. 3, 2005

Chu, Cordia Ming-Yeuk, 'Menstrual beliefs of Chinese women', *Journal of the Folklore Institute*, vol. 17, no. 1, 1980

Cibulka, Nancy J., 'Toxic shock syndrome and other tampon related risks', *The Journal of Obstetric, Gynaecologic and Neonatal Nursing*, vol. 12, no. 2, 1983

Collins, Rebecca, 'Concealing the poverty of traditional historiography: myth as mystification in historical discourse', *Rethinking History*, vol. 7, no. 3, 2003

Corner, George W., 'Our knowledge of the menstrual cycle, 1910–1950', *The Lancet*, vol. 257, no. 6661, 28 April 1951

Costos, Daryl; Ackerman, Ruthie and Paradis, Lisa, 'Recollections of menarche: communication between mother and daughter regarding menstruation', *Sex Roles*, vol. 46, nos 1/2, January 2002

Crawford, Patricia, 'Attitudes to menstruation in seventeenth-century England', *Past and Present*, vol. 91, no. 1, 1981

Crawfurd, Raymond, 'Notes on the superstitions of menstruation' *The Lancet*, vol. 186, no. 4816, 18 December 1915

Dahal, Khagendra, 'Nepalese woman dies after banishment to shed during menstruation', 'News', in *British Medical Journal*, vol. 337, 22 November, 2008

d'Arcangues, Catherine, 'WHO statement on hormonal contraception and bone health', *Contraception*, vol. 73, no. 5, 2006

Davalos, Karen Mary, '*La Quinceañera*: making gender and ethnic identities', *Frontiers: A Journal of Women's Studies*, vol. 16, nos 2/3 1966

Davis, Geoffrey, '"Menstrual toxin" and human fertility', *Lancet*, vol. 303, issue 7867, 8 June 1974

Dean-Jones, Lesley, 'Menstrual bleeding according to Hippocratics and Aristotle', *Transactions of the American Philological Association* vol. 119, 1989

Do Amaral, Maria Clara Estanislau, Hardy, Ellen, Hembling, Eliana Maria, Faúndes, Anibal, 'Menstruation and amenorrhea: opinion of Brazilian women', *Contraception*, vol. 72, no. 2, 2005

Douglas, Mary, 'Red Riding Hood: an interpretation from anthropology, *Folklore*, vol. 106, 1995

Drill, Victor A., 'History of the first oral contraceptive', *Journal of Toxicology and Environmental Health*, Part A, vol. 3, no 1, 1977

Ernster, Virginia L., 'Expectations about menstruation among premenarcheal girls', *Medical Anthropology Newsletter*, vol. 8, no. 4, 1977

Farrell-Beck, Jane, and Kidd, Laura Klosterman; 'The roles of health professionals in the development and dissemination of women's sanitary products, 1880–1940', *The Journal of the History of Medicine and Allied Sciences*, vol. 51, no. 3, 1996

Ferrero, Simone, Abbamonte, Luiza Helena, Giordano, Margherita, Alessandri, Franco, Anserini, Paola, Remorgida, Valentino, Ragni, Nicola, 'What is the desired menstrual frequency of women without menstrual-related symptoms?' *Contraception*, vol. 73, no. 5, 2006

Finn, Colin A., 'Why do women menstruate? Historical and evolutionary view', *European Journal of Obstetrics and Gynaecology and Reproductive Biology*, vol. 70, nos. 3–8, 1996

Freeman, William, and Looney, Joseph M., with the technical assistance of Rose R. Small, 'Studies on the phytotoxic index: II. menstrual toxin ("Menotoxin") from the Worcester State Hospital and the Memorial Foundation for Neuro-Endocrine Research Worcester, Massachusetts', *Journal of Pharmacological and Experimental Therapeutics*, vol. 52, no. 2, 1934

Furth, Charlotte; Shu-Yeuh, Ch'en, 'Chinese medicine and the anthropology of menstruation in contemporary Taiwan, *Medical Anthropology Quarterly*, vol. 6, no. 1, 1992

Garaud, Yolette, 'A student's journal: on menstruation', *Women's Studies Newsletter*, vol. 6, no. 3, 1978

Garg, Suneela, Sharma, Nandini, Sahay, Ragini, 'Socio-cultural aspects of menstruation in an urban slum in Delhi, India', *Reproductive Health Matters*, vol. 9, no. 17, 2001

Gillooly, Jessica B., 'Making menarche positive and powerful for both mother and daughter', *Women and Therapy*, vol. 27, no. 3, 2004

Golub, Sharon, Catalano, Joan, 'Recollections of menarche and women's subsequent experiences with menstruation', *Women and Health*, vol. 8, no. 1, 1983

Grieg, Alecia J., Palmer, Michelle A., Chepulis, Lynne M., 'Hormonal contraceptive practices in young Australian women (<25 years) and their possible impact on menstrual frequency and iron requirements', *Sexual and Reproductive Healthcare*, vol. 1, no. 3, 2010

Gunson, Jessica Shipman, '"More natural but less normal": reconsidering medicalisation and agency through women's accounts of menstrual suppression', *Social Science and Medicine*, vol. 71, no. 7, 2010

Gupta, A.K., Vatsayan, A., Ahluwalia, S.K., Sood, R.K., Mazta, S.R., Sharma, R., 'Age at menarche, menstrual knowledge and practice in the apple belt of Shimla hills', *Journal of Obstetrics and Gynaecology*, vol. 16, no. 6, 1996

Harrison, Lyn, '"It's a nice day for a white wedding": the debutante ball and constructions of Femininity', *Feminism and Psychology*, vol. 6, no. 4, 1997

Hartman, Tova; Marmon, Naomi, 'Lived regulations, systemic attributions: menstrual separation and ritual immersion in the experiences of Orthodox Jewish women', *Gender and Society*, vol. 18, no. 3, 2004

Helgerson, Steven D., 'Toxic-shock syndrome: tampons, toxins, and time: the evolution of understanding an illness', *Women and Health*, vol. 6, no. 3, 1981

Hicks, Caitlin W., and Rome, Ellen S., 'Menstrual manipulation: options for suppressing the cycle', *Cleveland Clinic Journal of Medicine*, vol. 77, no. 7, 2010

Hitchcock, Christine L., 'Elements of the menstrual suppression debate', *Healthcare for Women International*, vol. 29, no. 7, 2008

Hodes, Horace L., 'Progress in pediatrics: introduction to the presentation of the John Howland medal and award of the American Pediatric Society to Dr Bela Schick', *AMA American Journal of Diseases of Children*, vol. 89. no. 2, 1955

Holdrege, Barbara A., 'Body connections: Hindu discourses of the body and the study of religion', *International Journal of Hindu Studies*, vol. 2, no. 3, 1998

Hopkins, M. K., 'The age of Roman girls at marriage', *Population Studies*, vol. 18, no. 3, 1965

Johnston-Robledo, Ingrid; Barnack, Jessica; Wares, Stephanie, '"Kiss your period goodbye": menstrual suppression in the popular press', *Sex Roles*, vol. 54, nos. 5–6, 2006

Johnston-Robledo, Ingrid, Ball, Melissa, Lauta, Kimberley, and Zekoll, Ann, 'To bleed or not to bleed: young women's attitudes toward menstrual suppression', *Women and Health*, vol. 38, no. 3, 2010

Jones, Irene Heywood, 'Menstruation: the history of sanitary protection', *Nursing Times*, March 1980

Junod, Suzanne White, and Marks, Lara, 'Women's trials: the approval of the first oral contraceptive pill in the United States and Great Britain', *Journal of the History of Medicine and Allied Sciences*, vol. 57, no. 2, 2002

Kaunitz, Andrew M., 'Menstruation: choosing whether ... and when', *Contraception*, vol. 62, no. 6, 2000

Kemper, Steven, 'Time, person, and gender in Sinhalese astrology', *American Ethnologist*, Vol. 7, no. 4, 1980

Knudsen, Dean D., 'Socialization to elitism: a study of debutantes', *The Sociological Quarterly*, vol. 9, no. 3, 1968

Koff, Elissa, and Rierdan, Jill, 'Preparing girls for menstruation: recommendations from adolescent girls', *Adolescence*, vol. 30, no. 120, 1995

Koff, Elissa, Rierdan, Jill, and Sheingold, Karen, 'Memories of menarche: age, preparation, and prior knowledge as determinants of initial menstrual experience', *Journal of Youth and Adolescence*, vol. 11, no. 1, 1982

Laslett, Peter, 'Age at menarche in Europe since the eighteenth-century', *Journal of Interdisciplinary History*, vol. 2, no. 2, 1971

Lee, Janet, 'Menarche and the (hetero) sexualization of the female body', *Gender and Society*, vol. 8, no. 3, 1994

Lee, Janet, and Sasser-Coen, Jennifer, 'Memories of menarche: older women remember their first period', *Journal of Aging Studies*, vol. 10, no. 2, 1996

Liebling-Kalifani, Helen, Marshall, Angela, Ojiambo-Ochieng, Ruth, and Nassozi, Margaret Kakembo, 'Experiences of women war-torture survivors in Uganda: implications for health and human rights', *Journal of International Women's Studies*, vol. 8, no. 4, 2007

Logan, Deana Dorman, 'The menarche experience in twenty-three foreign countries', *Adolescence*, vol. 15, no. 58, 1980

Lord, Alexandra, '"The Great Arcana of the Deity": menstruation and menstrual disorders in eighteenth-century British medical thought', *Bulletin of the History of Medicine*, vol. 73, no. 1, 1999

Macht, David L., and Lubin, Dorothy S., 'A phyto-pharmacological study of menstrual toxin', *Journal of Pharmacology and Experimental Therapeutics*, vol. 22, no. 5, 1923

Mahon, Thérèse; Fernandes, Maria, 'Menstrual hygiene in South Asia: a neglected issue for WASH (water, sanitation and hygiene) programmes', *Gender and Development*, vol. 18, no. 1, 2010

Manderson, Lenore, 'Traditional food beliefs and critical life events in Peninsular Malaysia', *Social Science Information*, vol. 20, no. 6, 1981

Manniche, E., 'Age at menarche: Nicolai Edvard Ravn's data on 3385 women in mid-19th century Denmark', *Annals of Human Biology*, vol. 10, no. 1, 1983

Montgomery, Rita E., 'A cross-cultural study of menstruation, menstrual taboos, and related social variables', *Ethos*, vol. 2, no. 2, 1974

Moseley, Sophia, 'Practical protection', *Nursing Standard*, vol. 23, no. 6, 2008

Nawaz, Jamila, Lal, Shamma, Raza, Saira, and House, Sarah, 'Oxfam experience of providing screened toilet, bathing and menstruation units in its earthquake response in Pakistan', *Gender and Development*, vol. 18, no. 1, 2010

Neufeld, Christine, 'Speakerly women and scribal men', *Oral Tradition*, vol. 14, no. 2, 1999

Oram, Charlotte, and Beck, Judith, 'The tampon: investigated and challenged', *Women and Health*, vol. 6, no. 3, 1981

Orringer, Kelly and Gahagan, Sheila, 'Adolescent girls define menstruation: a multiethnic exploratory study', *Health Care for Women International*, vol. 31, no. 9, 2010

Oster, Emily and Thornton, Rebecca, 'Menstruation, sanitary products, and school attendance: evidence from a randomized evaluation', *American Economic Journal: Applied Economics*, vol. 3, no. 1, 2011

Patel, Kartikeya C., 'Women, earth, and the goddess: a Shākta-Hindu interpretation of embodied religion', *Hypatia*, vol. 9, no. 4, 1994

Phipps, William E., 'The menstrual taboo in the Judeo-Christian tradition, *Journal of Religion and Health*, vol. 19, no. 4, 1980

Pickles, Vernon R., "'Menstrual toxi'" again', *Lancet*, vol. 303, issue 7869, 22 June 1974

Pickles, Vernon R., 'Prostaglandins and dysmenorrhea: historical survey', *Acta Obstretrica et Gynecologia Scandanavia*, vol. 58, no. S87, 1979

Pillemer, David B., Koff, Elissa, Rhinehardt, Elizabeth D., Rierdan, Jill, 'Flashbulb memories of menarche and adult menstrual distress' *Journal of Adolescence*, vol. 10, no. 2, 1987

Posner, Rachel Blumstein 'Early menarche: a review of research on trends in timing, racial differences, etiology and psychosocial consequences', *Sex Roles*, vol. 54, nos 5–6, 2006

Post, J.B., 'Ages at menarche and menopause: some medieval authorities', *Population Studies*, vol. 25, no. 1, 1971

Powers, Marla N., 'Menstruation and reproduction: an Oglala case', *Signs*, vol. 6, no. 1, 1980

Read, Christine M., 'New regimes with combined oral contraceptive pills – moving away from traditional 21/7 cycles', *The European Journal of Contraception and Reproductive Health Care*, vol. 15, no. 2, 2010

Reid, Helen Evans, 'The brass-ring sign', *Lancet*, vol. 303, no. 7864, 18 May 1974

Rierdan, Jill and Koff, Elissa, 'Timing of menarche and initial menstrual experience', *Journal of Youth and Adolescence*, vol. 14, no. 3, 1985

Rierdan, Jill and Koff, Elissa, 'Preparing girls for menstruation: recommendations from adolescent girls', *Adolescence*, vol. 30, no. 120, 1995

Rose, Jennifer Gorman, Chrisler, Joan C., and Couture, Samantha, 'Young women's attitudes toward continuous use of oral contraceptives: the effect of priming positive attitudes toward menstruation on women's willingness to suppress menstruation', *Health Care for Women International*, vol. 29, no. 7, 2008

Roth, Nathan, 'The personalities of two pioneer medical women: Elizabeth Blackwell and Elizabeth Garrett Anderson', *Bulletin of the New York Academy of Medicine*, vol. 47, no. 1, 1971

Ruble, Diane N., and Brooks-Gunn, Jeanne, 'The experience of menarche' *Child Development*, vol. 53, no. 6, 1982

Sanabria, Emilia, 'The politics of menstrual suppression in Brazil', *Anthropology News*, vol. 50, no. 2, 2009

Sangren, P. Steven, 'Female gender in Chinese religious symbols: Kuan Yin, Ma Tsu, and the "eternal mother"', *Signs*, vol. 9, no. 1, 1983

Sanjakdar, Fida, "'Teacher talk": the problems, perspectives and possibilities of developing a comprehensive sexual health education curriculum for Australian Muslim students', *Sex Education*, vol. 9, no. 3, 2009

Sarkar, Tanika, 'A prehistory of rights: the age of consent debate in colonial Bengal', *Feminist Studies*, vol. 26, no. 3, 2000

Schlegel, Alice and Barry III, Herbert, 'Adolescent initiation ceremonies: a cross-cultural code', *Ethnology*, vol. 18, no. 2, 1979

Schlegel, Alice and Barry III, Herbert, 'The evolutionary significance of adolescent initiation ceremonies', *American Ethnologist*, vol. 7, no. 4, 1980

Schroeder, Fred E. H., 'Feminine hygiene, fashion and the emancipation of American women', *American Studies*, vol. 17, no. 2, 1976

Shail, Andrew, "'Although a woman's article": menstruant economics and creative waste', *Body and Society*, vol. 13, no. 4, 2007

Short, R. V., 'The evolution of human reproduction', *Proceedings of the Royal Society of London. Series B, Biological Sciences*, vol. 195, no. 1118, 1976

Skandhan, K.P., Pandya, Amita K., Skandhan, Sumangala, Mehta, Yagnesh B., 'Menarche: prior knowledge and experience', *Adolescence*, vol. 23, no. 89, 1988

Smith, Jane I., Haddad, Yvonne, 'Eve: Islamic image of woman', *Women's International Forum*, vol. 5, no. 2, 1982

Smith-Rosenberg, Carroll, 'Puberty to menopause: the cycle of femininity in nineteenth-century America', *Feminist Studies*, vol. 1, no. 3/4, 1973

Sniekers, Marijke, 'From little girl to young woman: the menarche ceremony in Fiji', *Fijian Studies*, vol. 3, no. 2, 2005

Sokol, B.J., '"Tilted Lees", dragons, haemony, menarche, spirit, and matter in Comus', *The Review of English Studies*, New Series, vol. 41, no. 163, 1990

Spellberg, D. A., 'Writing the unwritten life of the Islamic Eve: menstruation and the demonization of motherhood', *International Journal of Middle East Studies*, vol. 28, no. 3, 1996

Steinberg, Jonah, 'From a "Pot of Filth" to a "Hedge of Roses" (and back): changing theorizations of menstruation in Judaism', *Journal of Feminist Studies in Religion*, vol. 13, no. 2, 1997

Strange, Julie-Marie, 'Teaching menstrual etiquette in England, c. 1920s to 1960s', *Social History of Medicine*, vol. 14, no. 2, 2001

Tanner, J.M., Ellison, Peter T., Bullough, Vern L., 'Menarcheal age', *Science*, vol. 214, no. 4521, 1981

Teitelman, Anne M., 'Adolescent girls' perspectives of family interactions related to menarche and sexual health', *Qualitative Health Research*, vol. 14, no. 9, 2004

Thomas, Sarah L., Ellertson, Charlotte, 'Nuisance or natural and healthy: should monthly menstruation be optional for women?', *Lancet*, vol. 355, no. 9207, 11 March 2000

Thornton, Madeline 'The use of vaginal tampons for the absorption of menstrual discharges', *American Journal of Obstetrics and Gynaecology*, vol. 46, no. 2, 1943

Thurén, Britt-Marie, 'Opening doors and getting rid of shame: experiences of first menstruation in Valencia, Spain', *Women's Studies International Forum*, vol. 17, nos. 2–3, 2004

Trad, Paul V., 'Menarche: a crossroad that previews developmental change', *Contemporary Family Therapy*, vol. 15, no. 3, 1993

Trego, Lori L., and Jordan, Patricia J., 'Military women's attitudes toward menstruation and menstrual suppression in relation to the deployed environment', *Women's Health Issues*, vol. 20, no. 4, 2010

Uskul, Ayse K., 'Women's menarche stories from a multicultural sample', *Social Science and Medicine*, vol. 59, no. 4, 2004

Vertinsky, Patricia, 'Exercise, physical capability, and the eternally wounded woman in late nineteenth-century North America', *Journal of Sport History*, vol. 14, no. 1, 1987

Wardell, Diane Wind, and Czerwinski, Barbara, 'A military challenge to managing feminine and personal hygiene', *Journal of the American Academy of Nurse Practitioners*, vol. 13, no. 4, 2001

Weerasinghe, Chandrani, Karaliedde, Srikanthi, Wikramanayake, T. W., 'Food beliefs and practices among Sri Lankans: temporary food avoidances by women', *Journal of the National Science Council of Sri Lanka*, vol. 10, no. 1, 1982

Wiegratz, I; Hommel, H.H; Zimmermann, T; Kuhl, H. 'Attitude of German women and gynaecologists towards long-cycle treatment with oral contraceptives', *Contraception*, vol. 69, no. 1, 2004

Winslow, Deborah, 'Rituals of first menstruation in Sri Lanka', *Man*, vol. 15, no. 4, 1980

Wood, Charles T., 'The doctor's dilemma: sin, salvation and the menstrual cycle in medieval thought', *Speculum*, vol. 56, no. 4, 1981

Miscellaneous Papers and Monographs

Lynch, Pip, 'Menstrual waste in the backcountry', *Science for Conservation 35*, Department of Conservation, Wellington, 1996

'Product News', *Australian Pharmacist*, December 2012

Varina Tjon A. Ten, 'Menstrual Hygiene as a big taboo', *Menstrual Hygiene: a Neglected Condition for the Achievement of Several Millennium Development Goals*, European Commission – EuropeAid, Zoetermeer, 2007

World Health Organisation Western Pacific Region, 'Sexual and reproductive health of adolescents and youths in the Philippines: a review of literature and projects 1995–2003', Office of Publications, World Health Organisation, Geneva, 2005

Archival Records

Letter, Surgeon Superintendent Richard Eades, *Roman Emperor*, to the Secretary Colonial Land and Emigration Commissioners, Stephen Walcott, 25 October 1848, GRG 24/6/1848/1763, State Records of South Australia

Australian Bureau of Statistics

3301.0: Births, Australia 2009

Summary tables: 2.20: Births, Australia, selected years

www.abs.gov.au/ausstats/abs@nsf/Products/5ECFEOF9C48

Internet

Akhter, Saheen, 'Knowledge, attitudes and practices on reproductive health and rights of urban and rural women in Bangladesh', 2007, no publication details, http://kamome.lib.ynu.ac.jp/dspace/bitstream/10131/3157/1/3-131-Akhter.pdf

Aniebue, Uzochukwu Uzoma, Aniebue, Patricia Nonelum, Nwankwo, Theophilus Ogochukwu, 'The impact of pre-menarcheal training on menstrual practices and hygiene of Nigerian schoolgirls', *Pan African Medical Journal*, vol. 1, no. 2, 2009, www.panafrican-med-journal.com/content/article/2/9/full

Alliance for African Women's Initiative, 'Sexual maturation and menstrual management practices associated with schoolgirls in Ghana', 2010, http://afawigh.org/publication/sexual-maturation-and-menstrual-management-practices-associated-with-school-girls-in-ghana.html

Appel-Slingbaum, Caren at the Museum of Menstruation and Women's Health, 'The tradition of slapping our daughters', www.mum.org/slap.htm2000

Ahmed, Rokeya, and Yesmin, Kabita, 'Menstrual hygiene: breaking the silence', in *WaterAid Beyond Construction: a Collection of case Studies from Sanitation and Hygiene Promotion Practitioners in South Asia*, James Wicken, Joep Verhagen, Christine Sijbesma, Carmen da Silva, Peter Ryan (eds), WaterAid, London, 2008, www.wateraid.org/document/ch21_menstrual_hygiene_breaking_the_silence.pdf

Bharadwaj, Sowmyaa, and Patkar, Archana, 'Menstrual hygiene and management in developing countries: taking stock', Junction Social, Mumbai, 2004, 'BRAC sanitary napkins and birthing kits', www.mum.org/menhydev.htm

'Chronological Index of Patents Applied and Patents Granted 1863', www.archive.org/details.chronologicalin05offigoog

Clarke, Edward H., *Sex in Education; or, a Fair Chance for the Girls* (1873), James R. Osgood and Company, Boston, 1875. Project Gutenberg Literary Archive Foundation 2006, www.gutenberg.org/ebooks/18504

Darwin, Charles R., *The Descent of Man*, second edition revised and augmented, John Murray, London, 1874 http://darwin-online.org.uk/contents.html#descent

Del Giudice, Luisa, 'Wine makes good blood: wine culture among Toronto Italians', http://luisadg.org/wp/wp-content/uploads/2009/11/LGG-Cantina.PDF

'Depo Provera information sheet', Royal Women's Hospital Melbourne, www.thewomens.org.au/DepoProveraAContraceptiveInjection

Dickson, Scott, and Wood, Ruth, 'The perceptions, experiences and meanings rural girls ascribe to menarche: implications for teachers/teachers in training', paper presented at the Australian Association for Research in Education Conference, Hobart, 1995, www.aare.edu.au/95pap/dicks95021.txt

'Drugs and Supplements: Bromelain', www.nlm.nih.gov/medlineplus/print/druginfo/natural/patient-bromelain.html

'Dysmenorrhoea', *Patient Information*, Basildon and Thurrock University Hospitals, http://www.basildonandthurrock.nhs.uk

Gautam, Om, 'Is menstrual hygiene and management an issue for adolescent school girls in Nepal?', *Regional Conference on Appropriate Water Supply, Sanitation and Hygiene (WASH) Solutions for Informal Settlements and Marginalised Communities, Katmandu, Nepal, 19–21 May 2010* www.nec.edu.np/delphe/pdf/conference1.pdf#page=192

Hicks, Megan (curator), Powerhouse Museum Collection,'The Rags: Paraphernalia of Menstruation', http:// www.powerhousemuseum.com/rags

Hill, Mark, 'Müllerian duct', http://embryology.med.unsw.edu.au/notes/index/m.htm

'Judaism 101: a glossary of basic Jewish terms, concepts and practices', a project of the Union of Orthodox Jewish Congregations of America, www.ou.org

Maudsley, Henry, *Sex in Mind and in Education*, Hurst and Company, New York, 1884, www.archive.org/stream/sexinmindandine00maudgoog#page/n8/mode1up

Mooncup menstrual cup, http://www.mooncup.co.uk

Moreland City Council, 'Zero Waste for a Week Challenge', November 2010, http://www.moreland.vic.gov.au/environment-and-waste/rubbish-collection/zero-waste-challenge.html

'Prescribing information', *Seasonique*, www.seasonique.com/docs/prescribing-information.pdf, July 2010

Roberts, Alexander, Donaldson, James, Coxe, Arthur C., (trans.), *The Infancy Gospel of James* (1886), www.earlychristianwritings.com/text/infancyjames-roberts.html

Seymour, Kathryn, 'Bangladesh: tackling menstrual hygiene taboos', *Sanitation and Hygiene Case Study 10*, www.UNICEF.org/wash/files10_case_study_BANGLADESH_4web.pdf, 2008

Soucasaux, Nelson, 'Menstrual toxin: an old name for a real thing?', 2001, http://www.mum.org/menotox2.htm

Spencer, Herbert, *Education: Intellectual, Moral, and Physical*, Hurst and Company Publishers, New York, 1862, www.archive.org/stream/educationintelle00spenuoft#page/n297/mode/2up

Sztokman, Elena, 'Some rabbinic sources on women and Torah reading' compiled in honour of her daughter Avigayil's bat-mitzvah, 22 January 2005, http://www.shira.org.au/learn/read/

The Museum of Menstruation and Women's Health, http://www.mum.org/

Walt Disney Productions through the courtesy of Kotex Products, *The Story of Menstruation*, 1946, www.youtube.com/watch?v=bjIJZyoKRlg

Yaz Flex 'Public Summary' and 'Consumer Medicine Information', Therapeutic Goods
Administration (Aust), www.tga.gov.au/file/6491/download

Television

'Mazel Tov! Mazel Tov! Bar and Bat Mitzvah', *Compass*, ABC 1, Sunday 16 August, 2009

Booklets for Girls

Callender, Mary Pauline, *Marjorie May's Twelfth Birthday*, Australian Cellucotton
Products Pty. Ltd., Sydney, 1932

Kenny, Florence, *The Guide Through Girlhood*, Prof. Harvey Sutton (ed.), published by the
Father and Son Movement, Sydney, 1945

The Story Of Menstruation (1946), Kimberly-Clark Corporation, Lane Cove, NSW, 1953

As One Girl to Another, Australian Cellucotton Products Pty. Ltd., Sydney, 1949. No
publishing details given

Very Personally Yours, International Cellucotton Product Company, Chicago, Illinois,
1948. Published in Australia by the Education Department for Kimberly-Clark,
Lane Cove, NSW c. 1962

Growing Up and Liking It (1952), Johnson and Johnson Pacific Limited, c. 1968. No
publishing details given

Sharing Simple Facts: Useful Information About Menstrual Health and Hygiene, UNICEF
and Department of Drinking Water Supply, Ministry of Rural Development, New
Delhi, 2008

Newspaper Articles

The Age (Melbourne)

Webb, Carolyn, 'Christmas spirit knows no borders', 23 December 2010

Brady, Nicole, 'Puberty blues: the trials of young girls growing up faster than ever',
22 May 2011

Editorial, 'Tending to children with the bodies of women', 22 May 2011

The Argus

'Showing of sex education films', 23 February 1951

Daily Telegraph

Dunlevy, Sue, 'New Pill adds comfort for women', 25 September 2012

The Jakarta Post

Bone, Wendy, 'The magic "Jamu", part 1', 26 July 2009

The Mercury (Hobart)

'Lack of physical knowledge held harmful to young people', 14 January 1946

Sydney Morning Herald

Unknown author, 'Coming out, ready or not', 1 December 2004

Magazine Articles

Gare, Shelley, 'Secret women's business', *The Age Good Weekend*, 1 May 2010

Gladwell, Malcolm, 'John Rock's Error', *New Yorker Annals of Medicine*, 13 March 2000

Magazine Advertisements
The Australian Women's Weekly
'To women who love freedom' 29 March 1947
'Carefree', 26 September 1951; 26 March 1952
'The beach? Why yes! Any day for me' 26 March 1952

Newspaper Advertisements
www.trove.nla.gov.au
The Argus (Melbourne)
'Next time ... Kotex', 13 April 1928
'The poise of confidence', 'Woman's Magazine' supplement, 8 February 1941
'Carefree confidence', 'Woman's Magazine' supplement, 12 April 1941
'Spotlight confidence' 'Woman's Magazine' supplement, 13 September 1941
'Comfort is half the battle', 'Woman's Magazine' supplement, 21 March 1942
'Comfort is half the battle', 2 May 1942
'Priority for the women's services', 18 January 1943
'Can you date this fashion?' 2 March 1943
'Can you date this fashion?' 13 and 17 April 1943
'Why I switched to Meds by a nurse', 14 April 1943
'Why I switched to Meds by a school teacher', 21 April 1943
'Yesterday's fashions', 13 May 1943
'Fashions of the future', 13 March 1944
'Fashions of the future', 11 May 1944
'Accent on Freedom', 25 May 1946 and 20 December 1947
'Tampax is back', 'Woman's Magazine', supplement, 9 February 1947
'To women who love freedom', 'Woman's Magazine' supplement, 12 March 1947
'Make a date with freedom', 'Woman's Magazine' supplement, 16 April 1947
'To women of action ...', 'Woman's Magazine' supplement, 17 September 1947
'Modern women prefer Modess', 11 February 1948
'Beauty is not looks alone', 'Woman's Magazine' supplement, 1 June 1948
'Beauty has a better chance today', Woman's Magazine' supplement, 10 August 1948
'Go anywhere', 'Woman's Magazine', supplement 19 October 1948
'Gay and carefree is the modern miss', 'Woman's Magazine' supplement 21 December 1948
'More and yet more women are changing', 30 May 1954
The Brisbane Courier
'Announcing women's most intimate personal accessory', 16 February 1932
'To meet the requirements of the modern woman', 23 February 1932
'To meet the requirements of the modern woman', 1 March 1932
'To meet the requirements of the modern woman', 15 March 1932
'To meet the requirements of the modern woman' 26 April 1932
The Mercury (Hobart)
'At such times take care', 'Woman's Realm' supplement, 21 April 1937
'Mother dear – I need you so much!' 30 January 1940
'Modess shortage', 22 July 1942, 12 August 1942
'Supplies still limited', 13 November 1942
'Try it now', 27 November 1942
'Comfort, it's wonderful', 'Women's Realm', supplement 4 December 1942
'Accent on freedom', 27 February 1946

'You can go anywhere', 22 May 1946
'Free as the wind', 20 November 1946
'Free', *As One Girl to Another*, 11 March 1949
'Women who know are hard to please', 7 October 1950
'Comfort's the keynote', 5 April 1952
'Free', *Growing Up* 22 August 1952
'Just as important as the selection of a new season's gown', 29 October 1954
'Each year more and more women look forward to Holiday Time', 18 December 1954
Sun-Herald
'More Australian women buy Modess', 29 November 1953
Sydney Morning Herald
'…The Establishment of a highly efficient factory', *Sydney Morning Herald*, 20 February
     1931
'Not a shadow of doubt', 25 October 1947 and 11 November 1947
Coupon for *As One Girl to Another*, 2 July 1949
'Coming out, ready or not', 30 November 2004

Unpublished Journals

Dammery, Sally, 'Apache Puberty Ceremony, 1996', Mescalero Apache Reservation, New
     Mexico, USA

INDEX